"A wonderful guide for healers and their patients with cancer. It addresses the frustrations of many who argue that the treatment of cancer is worse than the disease. *Living Well with Cancer* allows one to get the most out of life while battling cancer."
—Mehmet Oz, M.D.,
director, Cardiac Assist Program, Columbia University,
author of *Healing from the Heart*

"This is one of the most reliable and thorough guides available for helping cancer patients and their families manage the ups and downs of cancer treatment. It can help anyone meet the challenges of cancer therapy, thus increasing its effectiveness."
—Larry Dossey, M.D.,
author of *Reinventing Medicine*

"Excellent . . . This seminal medical reference is the equivalent of the *What to Expect* series, providing patients with answers to the many questions they may not be able to ask their doctors. The authors encourage people to write a list of questions for their physician . . . then discuss the most common early stages—diagnosis, treatment options, clinical trials and treatment. The crux of the book is a detailed examination of common side effects such as hair loss and nausea, and less-known ones including heartburn, fever and hot flashes, followed by a discussion of medical and natural treatments. Finally, Moore and Schmais explain practical information such as hospice care, living wills and medical directives. While cancer patients obviously need to rely on a full complement of specialists, this volume is an excellent resource for both patients and their relatives or friends . . . Readers will learn that theirs is a shared experience, and that it's possible to limit the discomfort and pain that almost all cancer patients endure."   —*Publishers Weekly*

"[A] book that gets right down to practical, everyday, at-home management of symptoms, using readily available and noncontroversial remedies is surely a fresh and welcome addition to cancer literature."   —Joanna Bull,
founder and executive director of Gilda's Club

"Finally, I have seen how a thoughtful and fair presentation of different approaches to symptom management can actually work, and that the best of allopathic and holistic medicine can cohabitate. I applaud you both for tackling this controversial area of cancer care, and I look forward to having this book for both personal and professional reference."   —Susan Leigh, R.N.,
immediate past president of the
National Coalition for Cancer Survivorship

LIVING WELL
WITH CANCER

LIVING WELL
WITH CANCER

*A Nurse Tells You Everything
You Need to Know About
Managing the Side Effects
of Your Treatment*

KATEN MOORE, MSN, R.N., NP-C, AOCN
and
LIBBY SCHMAIS, MFA, MLS

A PERIGEE BOOK

A Perigee Book
Published by The Berkley Publishing Group
A division of Penguin Putnam Inc.
375 Hudson Street
New York, New York 10014

G. P. Putnam's Sons edition: April 2001
First Perigee edition: March 2002
Published simultaneously in Canada.

Perigee ISBN: 0-399-52751-6

Visit our website at www.penguinputnam.com

The Library of Congress has catalogued the
G. P. Putnam's Sons edition as follows:

Moore, Katen, date.
Living well with cancer : a nurse tells you everything you need to
know about managing the side effects of your treatment /
Katen Moore and Libby Schmais.
p.   cm.
Includes bibliographical references and index.
ISBN 0-399-14687-3
1. Cancer—Popular works.   2. Cancer—Treatment—
Complications—Treatment.   3. Cancer—Alternative treatment.
I. Schmais, Libby.
RC263.M574   2001   00-06237
362.1'96994—dc21

Printed in the United States of America

10 9 8 7 6 5 4 3 2 1

ACKNOWLEDGMENTS

THE AUTHORS WISH TO THANK ALL THE PEOPLE WHO HAVE educated and supported them during the researching and writing of this book, in particular all the clinicians we spoke with and all the people with cancer and other chronic diseases who allowed us to share their experiences and remedies. We would like to give a special thanks to Sam, Kevin, and Aurelia for their love, encouragement, and patience, and to Neeti Madan, Sheila Curry Oakes, and Joe Jacobs for their input and enthusiasm for this project. We couldn't have done this without each of you.

This book is dedicated to cancer survivors everywhere.
We want to thank you for all that we have learned
from you and honor you for your courage.

CONTENTS

FOREWORD

IT GOES WITHOUT SAYING THAT THE MOST EMOTIONALLY laden period in an individual's life is when the diagnosis of cancer is revealed. Most of us are ill prepared for the level of psychological and emotional stress that has to be endured. The sudden feeling of collapse consumes us at that instant as the words and meaning begin to sink in. As we recover from the suddenness of the news, we turn our attention to the hope of science to provide us with a cure. As the diagnosis of cancer or any other catastrophic illness moves from an abstraction to reality, we are faced with numerous questions on what to expect. The mundane issues are what most consume the cancer patient on a day-to-day basis.

As the first director of the Office of Alternative Medicine at the National Institutes of Health, I was frequently inundated with requests for information about alternative cancer therapies. In the years since I left that position, I have no reason to believe the demand has decreased for this type of information. Clearly, many individuals were seeking new cures, but many others were looking for practical solutions to many management issues confronting them on a daily basis. Therapeutic triumphs do not necessarily mean cure, but may come in the guise of a simple and practical solution to dealing with the side effects of a drug or how to cope with the stress and strain of pain and depression.

Katen Moore and Libby Schmais have created an excellent handbook for the cancer patient. They have identified and explored the issues not normally found in textbooks on cancer and often not easily explained by oncologists who concern themselves with addressing the main question: Will I be cured? They have provided practical solutions to the myriad of problems confronting the cancer patient and his/her family. It is a book that I clearly do not want to have to use. But if I do, I'm glad it's there.

—Dr. Joseph J. Jacobs,
first director, Office of Alternative Medicine,
National Institutes of Health

INTRODUCTION

By Sally Jenkins, co-author with Lance Armstrong
of It's Not About the Bike

Healing is an act of the imagination. It is equally a matter of common sense. The co-authors of this book are possessed of healthy doses of each, and they ask a seemingly simple question: why do we accept as a matter of course that cancer patients should suffer extraordinarily, and, what's more, that they must bear the suffering stoically, when something as simple as ginger ale might help? It's a question worth answering.

This book is a fortunate and much-needed combination of imagination and common sense, written by two friends who also understand both conventional and complementary medicines, and their practical applications. One of them, Katen Moore, is an oncology nurse whose formidable credentials are accompanied by an unconventional turn of mind. The other, Libby Schmais, is a novelist with two passions, writing and complementary remedies. The result of their partnership is *Living Well with Cancer,* a reference manual and an exercise in giving patients a new range of choices in the alleviation of their discomfort and a role in their own symptom management and cure.

Moore was in nursing school at The Institute of Health Professions Massachusetts General in Boston when she began to talk to patients about what they experienced during cancer treatments. She couldn't understand why some of their side effects couldn't be erased. One patient suffered from fear of potential nausea. "Well, what did your mother give you when you felt sick?" Moore asked.

"Ginger ale," the patient said.

The answer stayed with Moore. Ginger root, as it happens, actually has medicinal properties—it has even been studied for use in advanced Parkinson's disease. So there is a perfectly good reason why ginger ale is not only comforting, but genuinely useful in managing the side effects of cancer treatment. It occurred to Moore that there might be thousands of such examples, from flat cola to ice chips. Why, she wondered, should cancer patients be denied small comforts like these? One afternoon, her childhood friend Libby Schmais visited her in Boston. They sat in her garden and talked about their shared interest in complementary medicines, from the holistic to the homeopathic. They realized there was little or no literature on dealing with the side effects of cancer, much less a comprehensive guide, and they agreed that a book needed to be written. They began collecting anecdotes from cancer survivors.

Moore and Schmais were uniquely suited for the project. Moore has worked in many areas of cancer care, including chemotherapy administration, radiation nursing, palliative end of life care, and family counseling, and she was one of the first fifty fellows in the Leadership Development Institute of the Oncology Nursing Society in 1999. Schmais has worked as a medical researcher and has reviewed books for the Book of the Month Club for the past eight years. St. Martin's Press recently published her first novel.

Moore came to nursing late, but with the ardor of someone who had found her real calling. She had spent her twenties meandering through careers: she obtained an undergraduate degree in religion, she sang with a band in New York, she toured New Zealand for two months, she cooked in a restaurant in Cape Cod, and applied to law school. But the people she was closest to, among them her old friend Schmais, who she had known since she was eleven years old, wondered why she was pursuing law when what she really wanted to do was work with people who were "underserved and disadvantaged," as she put it. Nursing was the obvious choice.

In the midst of her training to become a nurse, Moore learned that an old friend was in Memorial Sloan Kettering, fighting leukemia. Moore made a trip to New York to donate platelets and found that her friend's chances weren't good. She was receiving massive amounts of blood products and was in need of a bone marrow transplant, but she had no family. Two siblings had died of HIV, her father had disappeared, and her mother refused to be tested. Moreover, her friend was given only a twenty percent chance of surviving the treatment. Not the disease. The *treatment*. The potential cure for cancer was as lethal as the disease itself. Moore never forgot that. It led her to oncology.

She sat up nights at Sloan Kettering with her friend, because she learned the nights were the loneliest and most terrifying times for a cancer patient. They talked about the symptoms, about the plaguing aches and pains and the emotional trapdoors that accompany cancer and its treatment. Moore discovered that the doctors and nurses attending her friend were so focused on trying to cure the disease that they tended to ignore the specific details of the suffering itself. If a patient felt ill, well, what else was to be expected? It was cancer after all. Patients were, albeit unintentionally, sometimes denied basic comfort and understanding.

It struck Moore that one of the most ordinary practical applications of medical care—to make someone feel better—wasn't applied to cancer patients. Why do we deny them the small things that might help? she asked herself.

As Moore's career as a nurse progressed—she joined Somerset Medical Center, a community hospital in Somerset, New Jersey—she stayed in touch with Schmais, who was working as a researcher and living in Astoria, New York. Together, they collected hundreds of anecdotes and small bits of information. Sorting through them was a challenge: not all complementary remedies worked, and some of them could be dangerous or counterproductive, especially in concert with conventional medicine.

The best information came from personal encounters with patients themselves. A man who was suffering from pancreatic cancer had heard that shark cartilage was a potential cure. He gulped bottles of the stuff—but he wouldn't eat. It posed a serious problem, because he needed food to maintain his metabolism.

A patient with breast cancer had terrible diarrhea, a side effect of one of the drugs she was taking. She was so miserable that she even considered halting treatment altogether. Moore asked that simple but curiously telling question: "What did your mother give you, and did it work?" The woman answered that her mother had routinely given her paregoric as a child, a tincture of opium that used to be sold over the counter, and it had worked for her. Opium is considered a last resort treatment, but in this case, the woman had had a good experience with it, so clinicians decided to try it. It worked like a charm.

Another woman with breast cancer experienced a facial rash, the effect of one of drugs she was taking. The rash was not debilitating, but it was itchy and unpleasant. Moore suggested cucumber: it's cooling and soothing, and used in facials. And it wouldn't create a problem in combination with her other medications. Again, it worked.

Moore and Schmais made a list of symptoms that they wanted to address, a list that they culled from the most frequently heard questions and complaints expressed by patients. They visited Gilda's Club in New York City, the national organization founded by comedienne Gilda Radner dedicated to providing and advocating wellness for cancer survivors. In numerous conversations, they learned firsthand what cancer survivors most want to know. What was there to do about hair loss, for instance? Schmais found this topic particularly engrossing and searched everywhere for answers to what might be useful. Vitamin E kept popping up, but unfortunately, she found that so far nothing has proven to be terribly effective. They heard about flower remedies, aromatherapy, and herbal teas. Cancer survivors want to know and try it all, from what teas to safely drink, to how to talk to family members. Above all, they want to know how to combine conventional medicine safely with complementary medicine.

But as Moore and Schmais collected information, they understood that some symptoms and side effects are so serious they shouldn't be managed. When it came to back pain, for instance, patients shouldn't ignore it or try to manage it on their own. Sometimes, they learned, pain has a purpose: to serve as an alarm.

Much recent cancer research is dedicated to finding remedies that won't wreak physiological havoc. It's an age-old dilemma for clinicians: how to find a cure for cancer that isn't as damaging as the disease itself. Many of the new treatments are exciting in this regard, and so are some of the emerging altnerative remedies. But just because a remedy is alternative or holistic, it doesn't necessarily mean it is gentler than conventional treatment.

As the work progressed, Moore and Schmais realized that there was a second category of side effects: the emotional ones. A major problem for cancer patients is the sensation that they are powerless and controlled by other forces, whether the illness itself or doctors and nurses. Moore and Schmais asked what they could do to give patients some control again. It seemed to them that a patient needed to feel that he or she was doing something on their own behalf. It might be important, for instance, to teach a patient how to manage their own medicines, to be able to administer some of their own care, so that they could feel some small bit of independence and feel that they still ran their own lives.

Moore and Schmais discerned that the emotional impact of the diagnosis could be as debilitating as the illness or the side effects of treatment. When the world has fallen apart, you need a way to put it all back together again. A very real challenge for Moore is to persuade patients that while it's a terrible and altering diagnosis, it's best dealt with actively. Those people who do best with the illness are those who make cancer a part of their lives, but who do not allow their lives to be completely defined by it. Example: a person receives a cancer diagnosis and stops everything. They soon feel sicker. They have halted all of their old familiar routines, the small comforting anchors of daily life. Illness takes over. No wonder they feel sicker.

Two of the most commonly asked questions in Moore and Schmais's experience are, what should I eat, and should I exercise? The answers, as usual, can be found in common sense. Fresh air and exercise are proven antidepressants. And we've known for a millennium that you need to eat your vegetables.

Finally, Moore and Schmais tried to consider perhaps the least examined and most mysterious part of cure: the mind. Clinicians can't say how much of cure is science, and how much is faith. But they do know for a fact that those who pursue treatment without belief have less chance of surviving. In other words, if you're convinced that ginger ale helps, it helps.

There are some things a cancer survivor can do to foster belief and cultivate an optimistic mind. Imagery and daydreaming may be helpful. Many cancer survivors told Moore and Schmais that they found a silver lining in a cancer diagnosis because it allowed them to discard old emotional luggage and problems that weighed them down and were relieved to reorder their priorities.

The very language we employ in discussing cancer might even be important. Can words be a factor in healing? Yes, the authors believe. It's important to understand that coping with health issues are hard, and to prepare yourself mentally for what's ahead, without becoming overly discouraged by the frightening terms in which it's discussed or overly optimistic. A doctor may tell a patient a chemotherapy regimen will be "easy," speaking comparatively, and the patient may then become discouraged to find it isn't "easy" at all. The fact is, chemotherapy is hard, by any standard. But to label chemotherapy "poison" and "toxic" doesn't help in getting through it either, and it may make you feel worse. Too often cancer is described as a "battle" or a "fight." These are harsh and discouraging terms for a process going on inside your body. The truth is that much has changed in cancer treatment: survival rates are higher, patients live a better quality of life than they used to, and they no longer die of the side effects. It's important to celebrate how far we've come.

Above all, knowledge has a powerful role in healing: the more educated a patient is about cancer, the better their chances. The more you can do to help yourself, the less power the diagnosis of cancer will have over you and your life.

Part One

A New Approach to Symptom Management

One

You and
This Book

WHILE MANY PEOPLE REACT TO A CANCER DIAGNOSIS AS an emergency, there are many people in the cancer community who believe it is helpful to approach cancer as you would a chronic disease such as diabetes or heart disease. Once you have a cancer diagnosis, you probably have already been living with the disease for a while, and you will continue to live with the disease. There can be crises in cancer that need to be addressed immediately, but generally speaking, you can continue to live your life and engage in many of your familiar activities while you are on cancer treatment.

Hopefully, after your cancer treatment is over, the cancer won't come back, and you will experience a lifelong remission. No one can accurately predict how long you will be cancer-free because, although you may have the same type of cancer as someone else, how it manifests in your body and how it responds to treatment varies from person to person. Statistics are based on groups of people similar to you in age, gender, disease stage, and treatment options. They are educated guesses, not absolute facts. Regardless of your prognosis, you can live meaningfully while you are on cancer treatment. Don't wait until treatment is done to live your life.

This is a guidebook for managing the side effects of cancer treatment. It can help you to live well despite the difficulties of treatment. In this book you will discover which side effects and symptoms to expect from cancer treatment, along with detailed descriptions of those side effects and symptoms. We let you know which complementary and conventional remedies are recommended for each problem, how to use them safely, and how to know when to get help from your cancer treatment team. We believe that the more options you have, the more able you will be to live well with cancer.

In this book you will find conventional medical recommendations to manage side effects, as well as complementary remedies. The complementary remedies we discuss include aromatherapy, acupuncture, bach flower remedies, herbal remedies, homeopathy, massage, meditation, nutrition, vitamins, therapeutic touch, and Yoga.

This book is not about treating cancer; it is about providing you with informed choices for managing the side effects and symptoms of cancer treatment and about helping answer your questions about what you can do for yourself. Can a special diet help you feel better? What fears do you have that you just can't discuss with your family? Your cousin tells you about an herb for depression he read about in a magazine article—is it safe for you to take while you are on treatment? Will a complementary remedy interfere with the effectiveness of your cancer treatment? What about aromatherapy? Or homeopathy?

This book presents information on using conventional and complementary remedies for cancer treatment symptoms. Despite the wealth of books written on ways to treat cancer and the many wonderful books on complementary therapies, there are very few books that combine these concepts. This book gives information on managing the problems of cancer treatment and specifically addresses the possible interactions complementary remedies may have with conventional cancer treatment and symptom management. These are important issues for cancer survivors.

This book is meant to be an aid to you. If something doesn't appeal to you, don't do it. We encourage you to do what feels right for you.

Don't let fear prevent you from deciding what feels right. It is your cancer and your body. Not everyone derives the same benefit from the same interventions. Even if you cannot entirely get rid of a problematic side effect, you may find a remedy that allows you to tolerate it well enough to live your life. We encourage you to keep trying different methods to find the one that works for you.

If you do not have a side effect or symptom that we describe here, don't worry. And don't think that you will suffer *every* side effect. We want you to know what can happen, but it won't necessarily happen to you.

Experiencing side effects doesn't mean that your treatment is not working. Nor will preventing the side effect negatively affect your treatment. Suffering does not make you stronger. It only interferes with your quality of life.

Life is full of simple pleasures and wonder. Let us help you live well and enjoy them.

> *This book is not meant to replace the therapeutic relationship you have with your clinicians. Don't be afraid to talk to your clinicians about your symptoms and side effects.*

Nine Simple Ways to Live Well with Cancer

1. Drink enough fluid every day.
2. Wash your hands thoroughly and often.
3. Let yourself have a bad day.
4. Communicate your needs.
5. Ask questions when you don't understand something.
6. Don't tough it out.
7. Eat.
8. Rest.
9. Enjoy yourself.

Two

YOU AND YOUR DIAGNOSIS

FACING A DIAGNOSIS OF CANCER CAN BE SCARY. YOU MAY BE feeling overwhelmed. You are probably imagining the worst-case scenario. You may even have trouble believing that this is happening to you. Your emotions are probably all over the place. Fear. Anger. Denial. All these reactions are completely understandable and completely normal. You have had a tremendous shock. Any emotion you feel right now is okay. There is no right way to feel, think, or behave. Whatever you are feeling, you are entitled to those feelings. If you are not ready to talk to people about your situation, that's okay, too.

Remember that getting cancer is not your fault.

FEARS ARE NOT REALITY

Fears are just that, fears. (See *Fear*, p. 225.) They do not have to become reality. Your imagination has the ability to create scenarios that are much worse than anything that can actually happen. We have all seen the fictional images of people dying of cancer in the movies and on television. Unfortunately, the Hollywood-type *Terms of Endearment* death scene is what we usually picture when we think of cancer. Please keep in mind that cancer diagnosis and treatment in the movies are used for their dramatic effect on the story; they don't reflect the experience of an average cancer survivor. Rarely do we get to see the millions of people who are living with cancer and who continue to live well with cancer.

What is true is that from the moment of your diagnosis, your life has changed irrevocably. Even if your cancer has been totally removed by surgery and you do not require any further treatment, you are now and forever a cancer survivor.

WHAT TO DO?

Try To Slow Down. You probably feel pressured to make immediate decisions about your treatment. While there are certainly rare situations and particular types of cancer where decisions need to be made rapidly, you usually can take time to gather the facts and think about your options. No matter what kind of cancer you have been diagnosed with, and no matter what your clinicians are telling you about how soon you should start treatment, take some time to think about your situation and discuss your options with loved ones. Except in the rarest cases—and your clinician will let you know if your situation is critical—a few hours or a few days will make no difference in how effective the treatment will be. It is important for you to take time to think about your options and know that you made the right decision for you.

COPING STYLES

People deal with the news of a cancer diagnosis in as many different ways as there are people. Some people shut down and pretend it isn't happening to them, while others become very motivated in searching out information about the diagnosis. Some people feel comfortable having their clinicians make most of the decisions, while other people want to be an active part of the decision-making process. There is no one right way to respond or act. You have to handle this situation in a way that works for you.

INFORMATION RESOURCES

There are many resources available to you. There is a wealth of information on the Internet, although it is important to find out the source and to confirm the authority of the information on the site. For the website addresses of the American Cancer Society, the National Cancer Institute, and the National Coalition for Cancer Survivorship, see the end of this chapter. There are also organizations dedicated to specific disease groups, such as The Leukemia and Lymphoma Society (www.leukemia.org) and various breast cancer groups, as well as hotlines you can call anonymously for information and support. To find disease-specific information, you will find a well-organized source of information at www.oncolink.upenn.edu/disease, a website sponsored by the University of Pennsylvania. Most cancer institutions also have websites.

> *Michael Lerner, in his excellent book* Choices in Healing, *makes the point that people put less care into their decisions about their cancer treatment than they would into buying a car. We encourage you to do things differently.*

SECOND OPINIONS

Don't ever be afraid to get a second opinion. Even if you trust your clinician absolutely, it is important that you feel totally confident with your diagnosis and treatment plan and have a good relationship with your clinician. It is also important that you get the best possible treatment available. Your clinician should be supportive of your decision to seek a second opinion. Remember that we are all human and mistakes do happen. You want to be sure of your options and your decisions in such a big event as a cancer diagnosis.

It is also completely reasonable to get a second opinion on the pathology report. This means that your biopsy specimens are sent to another pathology lab or are at least interpreted by a different pathologist at the same lab.

YOUR COMFORT IS PARAMOUNT

Be choosy about who will be working with you throughout this experience. You may need to ask around to find a clinician with whom you
feel really comfortable. If you think about it, you probably are already in
touch with a network of cancer experts. Through friends and relatives
and co-workers, you probably know someone who works in oncology or
someone who has already gone through cancer treatment. If you feel
comfortable talking about it, talk to the people you know and whose
opinions you trust to try to find the best clinician to meet your needs.

PREPARE YOURSELF FOR MAKING DECISIONS ABOUT YOUR CARE

If you can't think of anyone to talk to about your diagnosis, there are organizations that can help you. One such organization, the Cancer Hope
Network (see the end of this chapter) connects you with a volunteer
who has undergone a similar cancer experience to yours. You can ask
this person questions you may not be able to ask anyone else. This service is free and confidential.

KNOWLEDGE IS POWER

The unknown can be frightening. Many
people find reassurance in seeking out information about their diagnosis and their
treatment options. In one study looking
at reducing patient anxiety, patients were
given a tour of an oncology clinic and had
a question-and-answer session with an
oncology counselor. Afterward the participants reported that they experienced a
considerable reduction of their fears from
what they had felt beforehand. Learn

*Knowing the details of
your diagnosis and stag-
ing can make a big difference when your neighbor
starts volunteering all sorts
of awful stories about
someone else who had can-
cer. These people may be in
a very different situation
than you. As you know,
you can't compare apples
and oranges.*

what your comfort level is regarding information, and seek out what you need.

WHAT YOU NEED TO KNOW

Before you embark on your information-gathering journey, be sure to have certain information about your diagnosis, as the details can often be very meaningful in making decisions about your treatment options. It is a good idea to know the exact pathology of your diagnosis, that is, where in your body the biopsy was done and what was found. There is also pathology information that is called staging, which is based on how large the original tumor is, what kind of cells are found there, whether there is lymph node involvement, and if there is evidence of spread from the original tumor. There are a few different ways to stage cancer, and they are dependent on the type of cancer you have. For more specific information on staging, ask your clinician to explain the information in the pathology report to you.

> *What to bring to your consultation:*
> · *Any medical records you have*
> · *Any films and written reports (x-ray, MRI, ultrasound, CAT or CT scan, PET scan, venogram, arteriogram, etc.)*
> · *All current medications in their original bottles*
> · *Your insurance information*
> · *A notepad and pen and/or tape recorder*
> · *A friend or relative to help you remember what you wanted to ask and what was said.*

THE FIRST VISIT TO THE ONCOLOGIST

When you first go to the oncologist to discuss your treatment, it may be difficult for you to absorb all the information that is being thrown at you. It is a good idea to take someone with you to the consultation who can jot down notes of what is said to you for you to review later on. Another option is to tape-record the information. Try to write down your questions and concerns and bring them to your consultations. Don't be afraid to ask your clinicians all of your questions. No question is stupid, and you are not being a bother by asking questions. You are important, and your questions are valuable for your well-being. If your clinician gives you the impression that you are not allowed to ask questions, you may want to reevaluate your choice of clinician.

> Don't continue to see any clinician who makes you feel uncomfortable. Cancer and cancer treatment is hard enough without dreading every appointment.

Trust Your Instincts

If you don't feel comfortable with a clinician or if what he or she is suggesting doesn't seem right to you, you can take time to think about it. You can find a different clinician, do some research on your own, get a second or a third opinion.

CLINICAL TRIALS

Depending on the type of cancer you have been diagnosed with, and its staging, you will be offered at least a couple of treatment options, one of which is not to treat the cancer. For some cancers, there are fewer options than others. For almost every type of cancer, however, there is probably a clinical trial available at one institution or another. Your clinician may in fact be involved in one or more trials.

Very basically, there are three levels of clinical trials: phase I, phase II, and phase III.

Phase I

In a phase I trial, a drug is tested to see what is the highest dose of that drug that can be given before it reaches an unacceptable toxicity. Or a phase I trial can focus on how a particular drug should be administered (orally, intravenously, or by injection).

Phase II

A phase II trial is to learn how active an agent or procedure is against a tumor. A phase II trial provides information about how well the new drug or procedure works and generates more information about its safety and benefit. Each phase II study usually focuses on a particular type of cancer.

Phase III

A phase III trial is a head-to-head comparison of a standard therapy against a new therapy or agent. Phase III trials can involve large numbers of people and take place at different locations across the country. Be aware that these trials are randomized, so you do not get to pick whether you will get the new therapy or the standard therapy.

Clinical trials are conducted under specific guidelines called a protocol. The people entering the study have to fit the criteria of the protocol, and the clinical trial has to be conducted under specific guidelines to safeguard the safety of the participants and the accuracy of the results. Depending on your particular situation, you may have to look at a number of clinical trials before you find one where you meet the eligibility requirements.

For more information on clinical trials, please contact the National Cancer Institute. Their number is 1-800-4-CANCER, and at their website (http://cancertrials.nci.nih.gov) you can also search for more information on clinical trials.

DECISIONS ABOUT TREATMENT

One helpful way to think about clinical trials versus other treatment options is to think about who you are as a person. Are you a risk taker? Do you like to try new and daring activities? Or do you avoid risk? Thinking about how you make other decisions is a good way to make this one. For example, if you are someone who likes to gamble, a phase III clinical trial may be a good choice for you. This way the process of randomization of treatment is made for you. If you like to grab new opportunities and beat a new path, a phase II trial may be just right for you. If you are the type who likes minimal surprises and who likes statistical predictability, standard therapy may be your best choice. *Remember, your treatment is always your choice.*

SUPPORT GROUPS

After diagnosis is an excellent time to join a support group. An enormous event has just happened to you, and it can be very reassuring to talk to people going through similar experiences and having similar reactions. It may be difficult to make the first phone call to a support group or to ask for help, but it may be one of the most healing things you can do for yourself. There are general cancer support groups, groups specific to a particular disease, and support groups for the newly diagnosed. It may be more difficult to find a support group if you live in a rural area, but be sure to ask around about Internet-based or phone support groups. Or try to start one if you feel up to it; you may be surprised how rewarding it can be to start your own group. Another option is to see a professional counselor on your own.

RESOURCES

Diagnosis Cancer: Your Guide Through the First Few Months, by Wendy Schlessel Harpham (W. W. Norton, 1997).
Understanding Cancer: A Patient's Guide to Diagnosis, Prognosis and Treatment, by Norman Coleman (John Hopkins University Press, 1999).

To be matched with a support volunteer, you can reach the Cancer Hope Network at 1-877-HOPENET, or contact them online at www.cancerhopenetwork.org.

For information on how to set up your own support group, a good resource is the American Self-Help Clearinghouse, which you can reach at (201) 625-7101 for advice and publications.

National Coalition for Cancer Survivorship
426 C Street N.E.
Washington, D.C. 20002
(202) 544-1880
www.nccs.org

National Cancer Information Service
900 Rockville Pike
Bethesda, MD 20982
(800) 4-CANCER
cancernet.nci.nih.gov

American Cancer Society
www.cancer.org

COMPLEMENTARY THERAPIES

T HROUGHOUT THIS BOOK WE RECOMMEND A VARIETY OF remedies for cancer symptom management for adults. Because individual preferences vary greatly, we offer a few potential remedies for each symptom. A brief overview follows of the complementary therapies we mention extensively throughout the book. For each therapy, we give cautionary advice and provide sources for further information, including websites. If a particular therapy appeals to you, by all means find out more about it from other sources. In all cases, we recommend that you always consider safety issues and possible interactions between medications, whether conventional or complementary, before pursuing a new treatment approach.

When combining conventional and complementary therapies, we recommend that you add only one new remedy at a time so that if you have a reaction you will know what it is from and can stop using it.

ACUPUNCTURE

Acupuncture was developed in China more than two thousand years ago. Skilled acupuncturists can painlessly insert thin needles into certain points along invisible channels throughout the body called meridians. The needles are usually kept in place for less than one-half hour.

Acupuncture is relatively simple and has been shown to be quite effective for pain and stress relief. Acupuncture has few side effects, and the cost is usually low.

Safety Precautions

Only consult an acupuncturist who is properly licensed. Be sure to let your acupuncturist know about your cancer, and make sure the acupuncturist does not place needles in an identified tumor site. It is not advised to have acupuncture performed if you are neutropenic (have a low white blood cell count), thrombocytopenic (have a low platelet count), have recently started on anticoagulation therapy, or have an infection such as a cold or flu. Be sure to determine that the needles are new and used only once. We do not know the safety of acupuncture while on radiation treatment or for two days before and after chemotherapy treatment. To be on the safe side, we recommend that you avoid acupuncture at these times.

Insurance

Many private health insurance plans and HMO plans cover acupuncture services. Contact your insurance benefits office before you make your appointment to find out if acupuncture is covered under your plan.

For More Information

Practice standards for acupuncturists vary widely from state to state. The only national standard that exists is governed by the National Certification Commission for Acupuncture and Oriental Medicine (NCCAOM). You can contact the NCCAOM at (202) 232-1404 to receive a list of certified acupuncturists.

AROMATHERAPY

Aromatherapy is the use of highly concentrated essential oils to treat a variety of conditions. Essential oils are extracted from various parts of plants, generally through a process of steam distillation or cool pressing, making the aromas extremely concentrated. The amount of essential oil that can be extracted from a particular plant varies; rose oil, for example, will be much more expensive than lavender oil. How aromatherapy works is still being investigated. One theory is that the molecules of the essential oils trigger the release of neurotransmitters that induce relief. While there is not much data in the medical literature, what there is looks promising in terms of helping cancer patients with their symptoms.

It is important to buy good quality essential oils. A quality essential oil should contain only that single essence, not any other ingredients. While perfumed candles and bath oils are enjoyable, they do not necessarily contain essential oils, or they may contain impurities. Herbal teas are also quite different from aromatherapy oils. Since essential oils are highly concentrated, herbal teas and essential oils should not be used interchangeably. In fact, essential oils should not be ingested under any circumstance.

Some of the conditions commonly treated by aromatherapy oils are anxiety, insomnia, nausea, pain, and some skin conditions. Specific healing properties are attributed to each essential oil. There are many good books on aromatherapy; or you can visit a certified aromatherapist (see below) to get an individualized recommendation. Be aware that aromatherapy will most likely not be covered by insurance.

Using Aromatherapy

As with most complementary therapies, more aromatherapy oil is not necessarily better. Most practitioners recommend using only a few drops at a time with most methods. Some of the methods for using aromatherapy oils follow.

DIFFUSION

Diffusion is when you spray aromatherapy oils into the air. To make a spray mixture yourself, take ten drops of an essential oil and add up to seven tablespoonfuls of water. If you are not going to be using it right away, you can add one tablespoon of alcohol to preserve it. Shake the mixture together, pour into a small spray bottle, and spray into the air, as needed.

MASSAGE

You can buy an aromatherapy massage oil, but you can also make one yourself. To make a massage oil yourself, put several drops of aromatherapy oil into a base oil, such as almond or jojoba.

BATHING

It is recommended that you use no more than eight drops of essential oil for an aromatic bath. You can also add between three and six drops of essential oil to a footbath or a Jacuzzi.

Safety Precautions

Aromatherapy oils are concentrated and should never be ingested internally, and they should not be used undiluted on the skin. If you have skin allergies or asthma, you may want to avoid aromatherapy oils. It is important to buy essential oils from a reputable source. We also do not recommend most aromatherapy candles; they are often scented with synthetic fragrances, and they can even emit harmful pollutants into the air you are breathing.

Insurance

Most private health insurance plans and HMOs do not cover aromatherapy services. Contact your insurance benefits office before you make your appointment to find out if aromatherapy is covered under your plan.

For More Information

To get more information or locate an aromatherapy professional in your area, contact the following associations:

American Alliance of Aromatherapy
PO Box 750428
Petaluma, CA 94975-0428
(707) 778-6762

American Aromatherapy Association
PO Box 3679
South Pasadena, CA 91031
(818) 457-1742
www.aromaweb.com

BACH FLOWER REMEDIES

Bach Flower Remedies were developed in the early 1900s by Dr. Edward Bach, a homeopathic physician in England. His belief was that negative emotional states underlie physical problems. Instead of treating an illness or symptom directly, these remedies are designed to relieve unwanted emotional states, such as despair or lack of confidence. The thirty-eight remedies begin as concentrated solutions made from flowers. These flower essences are then diluted and preserved in brandy, then again diluted with water. The theory is that although the flower remedies are extremely dilute, the therapeutic essence of the flower remains in each remedy. There is also a combination homeopathic remedy, Rescue Remedy, which is a combination of five flower essences and is used to cope with shocking or traumatic events.

Using Bach Flower Remedies

Bach Flower Remedies come in small bottles with droppers, and the usual dosage is a few drops of the remedy, either taken under your tongue or mixed with a little water and taken as a drink.

Safety Precautions

While there is brandy in the remedies, it is in extremely diluted form. However, if you are a recovering alcoholic or cannot have products containing alcohol or fermentation, you may want to avoid these remedies. Like homeopathic remedies, Bach Flower Remedies should work in a day or two, or you should try another type of remedy.

Insurance

We doubt that Bach Flower Remedies are covered by any insurance plan. However, you may contact your insurance benefits office to learn if this treatment is covered under your plan.

For More Information

To find out more about the flower remedies and for a list of practitioners, contact the Dr. Edward Bach Centre and Foundation at www.bach-centre.com or

> Dr. Edward Bach Foundation
> The Bach Centre
> Mount Vernon
> Bakers Lane, Sotwell
> Oxon, OX10 0PZ, UK
> Telephone: +44 (0) 1491 834678
> Fax: +44 (0) 1491 825022

CHINESE MEDICINE

One of the major assumptions of Chinese medicine is that illness is due to an imbalance of yin and yang and that by treating this imbalance and returning to a state of equilibrium, one can treat the illness. Chinese medicine is a very complicated system of medicine that has been used successfully for centuries. In this book we have neither the space nor the knowledge to go into an in-depth discussion of it. We do discuss acupuncture throughout the book and some Chinese mushrooms in the *Immunity* section of chapter 5.

Using Chinese Medicine

If you are interested in Chinese medicine, we highly recommend that you see a specialist in this ancient tradition. Another issue to keep in mind is that Chinese medicine is an entire system of medicine, as is Ayurvedic medicine from India, and it was not designed to be a complementary system to Western (or allopathic) medicine.

For More Information

You can find more information about Chinese medicine through the American Association of Acupuncture and Oriental Medicine, located in Pennsylvania, at (610) 266-1433 or on the website www.acupuncture.com.

HERBAL REMEDIES

Currently, in the United States, there is an enormous interest in medicinal herbs. In many rural communities in the United States alone, including the Amish, Appalachian, Cajun, and Shaker communities, herbal remedies have been used for centuries and are even prescribed by clinicians and healers for various symptoms and illnesses. In addition, many of the common remedies we use, such as aspirin and decongestants, were originally derived from what we now refer to as herbal remedies. We realize that there is conflicting information available about herbs and it can be hard to sort out the useful from the fanciful. We encourage you to find out as much as you can about the herb or remedy you are interested in (by consulting books and other resources) and to be discriminating in your choices. We also encourage you to talk to your clinicians and let them know what herbs you are taking or thinking of taking, as there can be interactions between herbs and allopathic medication.

Using Herbs

Herbs come in many forms, including capsules, tablets, extracts (liquid form), and teas, as well as in ointments and creams. Be aware that the herbs in food may also have medicinal effects. For example, garlic acts as a mild anticoagulant (similar to aspirin), so it is recommended that you avoid eating a lot of it for a few days before surgery.

Safety Precautions

It is very important to remember that herbs are medicines. Just because a plant or herb is called "natural" doesn't mean it is safe for you. Because of the current lack of regulation in the United States, it is especially important when using herbal medications to read the labels carefully and make sure that only the individual herb you are looking for is present and in the dosage you require. As with all remedies, more is not better. It is also extremely important to buy herbs from a reputable manufacturer. The herbs used for flavor in cooking are generally at nontherapeutic levels, and you should not be concerned about potential interactions of your cancer treatment with flavorful food.

It is also very important to have the correct name of the herb. As in the case of prescription medications, there are many similarly named herbs. Be aware of what you are taking, as the wrong herb could be harmful.

Unlike prescription or over-the-counter medications made by pharmaceutical companies in the United States, the manufacture of herbs and other food supplements is not regulated, although there is a movement toward having this kind of regulation. As of this writing, herbal products are not regulated by the FDA unless there has been a serious concern about safety due to deaths attributed to the product, as with herbs like ephedra (also known as ma huang) and comfrey.

Insurance

We doubt that herbal remedies are covered by most insurance plans. However, you may contact your insurance benefits office to learn if this treatment is covered under your plan.

For More Information

One reliable source of information on herbs is the American Botanical Council, which has a website at www.herbalgram.org. Another source of information is www.consumerlab.com, where you can find product reviews of individual herbs and supplements.

IBIDS DATABASE

If you are interested in doing your own research into the latest scientific developments regarding herbal medicine, you can search the International Bibliographic Information on Dietary Supplements (IBIDS) database, a service provided by the National Institutes of Health. This database contains published scientific literature on dietary supplements, including vitamins, minerals, and herbs. The website is located at http://odp.od.nih.gov/ods/databases/ibids.html.

HOMEOPATHY

Homeopathy was invented by a German physician, Samuel Hahnemann (1755–1843). The term *homeopathy* comes from a combination of the Greek words *homios,* "similar," and *pathos,* "suffering." Hahnemann was not only the inventor of homeopathy but was the first physician to try to prove his theory of healing through a series of what he called "provings," what we would now call clinical trials. The "law of similars" is one of the basic principles of homeopathy. Its basis is that small amounts of the substances believed to cause illness are used to treat that illness. Another principle, called the "law of infinitesimals," explains the method of homeopathic dosing. A typical remedy of 6x (x represents the Roman numeral 10) is one where a substance is repeatedly diluted in a one-to-ten dilution, repeated six times. After each dilution, the mixture is vigorously shaken. Some homeopathic remedies are so dilute that often no molecules of the healing substance actually remain in the solution. This is one reason that many practitioners of allopathic medicine find it difficult to give credence to homeopathy. However, Hahnemann's theory is that the solutions hold a trace memory of the original substance and therefore still trigger the body's immune response to the infection.

Another tenet of homeopathy is to match the remedy to the temperament of the individual, not merely to treat the outward symptoms of disease. Some of the more famous proponents of homeopathy were Daniel Webster, Louisa May Alcott, William James, W. B. Yeats, Charles Dickens, Benjamin Disraeli, and Pope Pius X.

Using Homeopathy

While you will find homeopathic remedies in various strengths, the more highly diluted (30x) is considered more potent than the less highly diluted (6x). It is recommended that you start out with the less diluted substance, for example, the 6x or 15x rather than the 30x.

Safety Precautions

Since many mainstream allopathic researchers and clinicians consider homeopathy useless and therefore harmless, there is not much information on the safety of homeopathy. However, homeopathic practitioners generally recommend that you use a homeopathic remedy only for a day or two, and if it is not working, discontinue it. It is also important to make sure that the remedy you are using fits your individual symptoms. If you are interested in homeopathy, we highly recommend that you see a homeopathic practitioner for consultation.

Insurance

We doubt that homeopathic remedies are covered by any insurance plan. However, you may contact your insurance benefits office to learn if this treatment is covered under your plan.

For More Information

To receive a directory of trained homeopaths as well as an information package on homeopathy, send $10 to the National Center for Homeopathy, 801 North Fairfax Street, Suite 306, Alexandria, VA 22314, or use their directory online at www.homeopathic.org.

MAGNET THERAPY

This controversial form of therapy is used for muscle, nerve, and joint pain. Although researchers do not know exactly how magnets work, in a recent study at Baylor Medical School in Houston, magnets were shown to be effective in reducing foot pain related to postpolio syndrome in diabetics. A study of magnets for relief of fibromyalgia pain is under way at the University of Virginia. While more research on the effectiveness of magnets in relieving various types of pain needs to be done, the current recommendations are to use magnets with strengths of between 300 and 5000 gauss (slightly stronger than your basic refrigerator magnet). Typically, people do not feel any direct sensation from the magnets.

Using Magnets

Magnets come in different shapes and sizes. They can be inserted in your shoes, seat cushions, and mattress pads. Small magnetic discs can be taped to the body in the area of discomfort. There is no certification of practitioners of magnet therapy, but some pain management clinicians are experienced and interested in this area. Magnets are available over the counter in health food stores and pharmacies. When purchasing magnets, we recommend you make sure they are from a reputable medical vendor and that the strength of the individual magnet is indicated on the label.

Safety Precautions

People with a cardiac pacemakers, defibrillators, low platelets, or bleeding disorders should not use magnets. For others, magnets with a strength of 300–500 gauss are considered safe to use.

Insurance

We doubt that magnetic remedies are covered by any insurance plan. However, you may contact your insurance benefits office to learn if this treatment is covered under your plan.

For More Information

Bio-Electro-Magnetics Insitute
2490 West Moana Lane
Reno, NV 89509-3936
(702) 827-9099

MASSAGE THERAPY

Massage has been used for centuries by different healing traditions all over the world to treat pain, relieve stress, and correct imbalance. By applying pressure and movement to the soft tissue, massage helps to stretch muscles, promote blood and lymph flow, and stimulate the nervous system. Massage has also been used successfully to treat complications of lymphedema and postoperative pain. Massage can also be used with aromatherapy for additional benefits.

Using Massage

There are many different types of massage. The one we recommend to a beginner is the gentle Swedish massage, which primarily consists of slow rhythmic strokes in the direction of the heart. Self-massage techniques are also helpful and can be easily practiced on the hands and feet.

Safety Precautions

Do not have tumor or metastasis sites massaged. As with any therapy, stop if you feel uncomfortable. Massage may cause a moment of discomfort as tight muscles release, but pain is usually a warning sign that should not be ignored. Communicate openly with your massage therapist about your diagnosis and treatment and about how the massage feels. Massage is not recommended for anyone with a rash or unhealed wound.

Insurance

Some private insurance plans and HMOs cover therapeutic massage. We suggest you contact your insurance benefits office before your appointment to learn if this treatment is covered under your plan.

For More Information

You can find a certified massage therapist from an organization such as the American Massage Therapists Association (AMTA) through their Find a Massage Therapist Locator Service at their website, www.amta-massage.org, or by contacting them at:

AMTA
820 Davis Street
Suite 100
Evanston, IL 60201
(847) 864-0123

LICENSING

Twenty-nine states currently regulate massage therapists. The National Certification Board for Therapeutic Massage and Bodywork administers the certification exam required to practice in these states.

MEDITATION

Meditation is a way of quieting your mind and can be used to cope with stress and anxiety. Meditation has also been shown, through numerous studies, to reduce high blood pressure and relieve chronic pain. Through meditation you can learn to focus your awareness.

Using Meditation

There are many approaches to meditation. Some are connected to spiritual practices while others are not. *Transcendental meditation* (TM) is one of the most common forms of meditation. It involves the repetition of a word called a mantra. This mantra can be any word: peace, love, Rama (the Hindu word for God), or any word or sound that has special meaning to you. *Mindfulness meditation* is another form of meditation, in which you learn to focus on the present moment. *Breath meditation* is yet another technique in which you focus on the process of slowly inhaling and exhaling.

Safety Precautions

There are no known special precautions to practicing meditation. However, meditation can bring up strong emotions. If you find meditation has a counterproductive effect on you, making you feel more anxious or uncomfortable, don't force yourself to continue.

Insurance

Some private insurance plans and HMOs cover meditation classes. Contact your insurance benefits office to learn if this treatment is covered under your plan.

For More Information

Insight Meditation Society
1230 Pleasant Street
Barre, MA 01005
(508) 355-4378
www.dharma.org

There are many excellent books and audio and video tapes on meditation, including:

How to Meditate: A Guide to Self-Discovery, by Lawrence LeShan (Bantam Books, 1984).
Breath Sweeps Mind: A First Guide to Meditation Practice, edited by Jean Smith (Riverhead Books, 1998).

THERAPEUTIC TOUCH

Therapeutic Touch is a process where the certified practitioner (often a nurse) moves his or her hands a few inches above the patient to redirect energy for healing. Despite the name, Therapeutic Touch treatments are generally done without direct physical contact between the practitioner and the patient. Therapeutic Touch treatments can increase a sense of well-being and decrease pain in persons with cancer. A typical Therapeutic Touch session lasts somewhere between ten and thirty minutes, during which the recipient sits or lies down fully clothed. The vast majority of patients who participate in Therapeutic Touch report feeling deeply relaxed during the treatment.

Using Therapeutic Touch

We suggest choosing a practitioner who has completed a training program in Therapeutic Touch and has several years of experience. There is no certification procedure. Nurse Healers (see below) offers a list of practitioners of Therapeutic Touch who belong to their association.

Safety Precautions

There are no medical conditions we know of that preclude Therapeutic Touch treatments. However, do inform your practitioner of the location of any tumor sites, as this can affect the treatment.

Insurance

We recommend you contact your insurance benefits office to learn if Therapeutic Touch is covered under your plan.

For Further Information

Nurse Healers Professional Associates
1211 Locust Street
Philadelphia, PA 19107
(212) 545-8079
www.therapeutic-touch.org

BOOK

Therapeutic Touch, by Dolores K. Krieger (Simon and Schuster, 1994).

VITAMINS AND MINERALS

Vitamins and minerals are generally absorbed from what we eat. Although only small amounts of most vitamins are needed, vitamins are necessary to health and well-being. Vitamins fall into two groups, water-soluble and fat-soluble. Water-soluble vitamins cannot be stored in the body, so they need to be taken daily, either absorbed from food or taken in a supplement form. Water-soluble vitamins include vitamin C and most of the B vitamins. Fat-soluble vitamins can be stored in the body for longer periods of time; they include vitamins A, D, E, K, and folic acid. Vitamins and minerals often serve specific functions once absorbed in our body; for example, vitamin K is needed for clotting, and calcium is needed for healthy bones and teeth. For more information on the specific nutritional needs while on treatment, see *Nutrition,* p. 244.

Using Vitamins and Minerals

RDAs (RECOMMENDED DAILY ALLOWANCES)

You have probably heard of the RDAs, and you can find them listed on foods and vitamin bottle labels. These guidelines were originally established by the federal government to determine the minimum amount of vitamins and minerals one would need to prevent once-prevalent nutritional diseases such as scurvy and beriberi. Be aware that the RDAs are guidelines intended for public health and they don't take into account the special nutritional needs of a particular person. For example, smokers and drinkers may become deficient in certain vitamins because alcohol and tobacco use can affect vitamin absorption. People under stress, the elderly, and the chronically ill also have different nutritional needs for similar reasons. Many researchers in nutrition and complementary health practitioners believe that following the RDA guidelines strictly will leave most of us lacking in certain nutrients.

Safety Precautions

As with any medication or remedy, more is not better. If you are going to take anything other than a daily multivitamin, we recommend that you consult a registered nutritionist or dietician for guidelines. When taking vitamins, take the recommended dose. We do not recommend megadoses of vitamins for anyone.

Insurance

Most insurance plans cover referrals to registered nutritionists and dieticians. Contact your insurance plan for specifics on how to receive this benefit.

For Further Information

If you are interested in finding out more about vitamins, you can find many excellent books on nutrition and cancer at your local bookstore or library or through various sources on the Internet. We also strongly urge you to consider requesting the assistance of a nutritionist experienced in cancer nutrition to evaluate your diet and make recommendations regarding vitamins and diet based on your individual nutritional needs and food preferences.

IBIDs DATABASE

If you are interested in doing your own research into the latest scientific developments regarding vitamins and minerals, you can search the IBIDs database, a service provided by the National Institutes of Health. This database contains published scientific literature on dietary supplements, including vitamins, minerals, and herbs. The website is located at http://odp.od.nih.gov/ods/databases/ibids.html.

YOGA

The word *yoga* is derived from the Sanskrit word for "union." The ancient practice of yoga has been used to lower blood pressure, increase relaxation, improve breathing, and maintain good flexibility and overall health and well-being. Yoga is generally taught in classes, although you can certainly learn it on your own from a video or book. A typical yoga session generally includes three parts: breathing exercises, a series of positions called asanas, and a brief meditation. Some classes also include chanting.

Using Yoga

Although you can learn yoga on your own from a video or book, we recommend taking a class so you can learn the proper basic techniques of yoga before you start practicing on your own. There are several different types of yoga, and some are quite athletic. Find out about the style and level of a yoga class before taking it. We recommend you start at a beginning level.

Insurance

Some private insurance plans and HMOs cover yoga classes. We suggest you contact your insurance benefits office to find out if this is covered under your plan.

Safety Precautions

If you've had a recent back injury or surgery, check with your clinician first before practicing yoga positions. Even if you can't do the postures, the breathing exercises and meditation practices may be very helpful. If you are taking a yoga class and there are any postures you find uncomfortable, feel free to modify them or rest on your back until the class goes on to the next exercise. It's a good idea to observe a yoga class before you try it to see if it's the level and style that is right for you. Prior to taking a class, let the instructor know any physical limitations you may have.

For More Information

American Yoga Association
PO Box 19986
Sarasota, FL 34276
(941) 927-4977
www.members.aol.com/amyogaassn

A good place to buy yoga tapes, books, and accessories is the website of the magazine *Yoga Journal* at www.yogajournal.com.

Part Two

REMEDY GUIDE

Four

SYMPTOMS AND REMEDIES

THE SYMPTOMS LISTED HERE ARE THOSE MOST COMMONLY experienced by people undergoing treatment for cancer. Sometimes these symptoms are related to the cancer itself, and sometimes they are a result of the treatment regimen. Remember, any new symptom is worth mentioning to your clinician in case it requires something more than self-treatment.

ACHES AND PAINS

Aches and pains are part of everyday life, but when you have certain cancers and are on specific treatments, aches and pains can be indicators of more significant problems. Certain types of aches and pains require a clinician's immediate attention, whereas others can be self-treated. However, always remember to be careful about combining different remedies for pain relief if you are on cancer treatment.

For nerve pain or burning, see *Numbness and Tingling,* p. 181.

For chronic pain related to your cancer, see *Cancer Pain,* p. 69.

Questions To Ask with New Pain

Is this a new or a different pain? When did the pain start and what were you doing? Try to describe it. Is it constant, intermittent, sharp, dull, throbbing, or tingly? What makes it worse? What relieves it? What does this pain prevent you from doing? Have you had similar pain in the past? What helped to relieve the pain then?

Knowing the answers to these questions will help you understand what is happening and communicate with your clinician. You may wish to write down what you feel so you will remember it when you are in the clinician's office.

DIAGNOSIS AND TREATMENT CONSIDERATIONS

If you are experiencing a new ache or pain that involves your back, hip, ribs, shoulder, arm, or leg, call your clinician.

Surgery

You should expect to feel some pain or discomfort while recovering from surgery. This discomfort is usually the worst for a day or two after surgery and then starts to improve as you start moving around and eating more. How long you take to heal depends on what type of surgery you had. Remember, your body needs time as well as good nutrition to heal. In most cases, you will have also been given prescriptions for pain medication or information on what to take for pain. Don't be afraid to take pain medications if you are experiencing discomfort. It is important to get up and move around after surgery. Taking pain medications will help you do this.

After surgery, you may need to adapt your movements temporarily to avoid discomfort. For example, after abdominal surgery, you may need to learn to get out of bed in a different way while you heal. Certain types of surgical dressings and supports (such as a girdle or elastic brace) can allow you more freedom of movement. For recommendations, discuss these possibilities with your surgeon or ask for a visiting nurse referral.

SURGICAL SCARS

The tingling, numb feeling of new surgical scars can last for months after the surgery and most likely will not be permanent. This feeling may be the result of the nerves in the skin waking up after having been disturbed by the surgery and suture process. While this sensation is annoying, it is probably better to leave the scars alone to heal. You can, however, gently massage and stretch the area of skin involved.

Chemotherapy and Biological Response Modifiers

PACLITAXEL (TAXOL), ETOPOSIDE (VP 16), TENIPOSIDE, VINCRISTINE (ONCOVIN), VINDESINE, INTERLEUKINS, AND INTERFERON ALPHA (ROFERON, INTRON A)

These medications have all been associated with the side effects of joint swelling, aches, numbness, and tingling. These side effects can happen even months after you have completed treatment. Inform your clinician if you have any of these side effects during or after chemotherapy treatment. See *Numbness and Tingling*, p. 181, for more on this topic.

RITUXIMAB (RITUXAN)

Rituximab (Rituxan), a monoclonal antibody used for lymphoma, has been reported to trigger pain in lymph node areas during the medication infusion (groin, underarms, neck, etc.).

FILGRASTIM (NEUPOGEN) AND OPRELVEKIN (NEUMEGA)

Filgrastim is used to boost your white blood cell count, and oprelvekin is used to increase your platelet production. Both can trigger bone pain because they stimulate bone marrow. This pain is usually experienced in the bones of the thighs, pelvis, back, ribs, and sternum. The actual injections of these medications can sting, but this is only an immediate sensation.

Antiemetics

Granisetron (Kytril), Ondansetron (Zofran), and Dolasetron (Anzemet) are medications used to prevent and manage nausea; they can all cause headaches.

Radiation

Some people report achiness when getting radiation that includes certain bones (usually the thigh bone, upper arm, scapula, pelvis, or ribs). You can take an analgesic such as acetaminophen (Tylenol) or ask your clinician to recommend something else for relief. Radiation can also cause discomfort by irritating the skin within the radiation field, sometimes severely.

Prevention

Relaxation techniques can help relieve everyday tension. Remember that these exercises take practice; the more you do them, the better they work. Try not to give up after only a few tries. Just the act of sitting still and breathing deeply can reap great benefits, even if you can only do it for a few minutes.

Don't forget the nonpharmacologic approaches to pain management. See Meditation, *p. 242, and* Relaxation, *p.252.*

While you are on treatment, even if you feel wonderful, now is not the time to begin training for the local marathon or to play contact sports. Preserve and cherish your well-being. If you have access to a pool, swimming is about the safest exercise you can do, but be careful to stay warm enough. Make a point to use sunscreen whenever you are out in the sun. And cover up to prevent too much sun exposure, even if it's warm outside.

Try yoga, deep breathing, gentle exercise, and stretching.

If you believe a medication is causing you pain, ask your clinician if you can switch to a different formulation. For instance, if the antinausea medication granisetron gives you a headache, try ondansetron or dolasetron next time.

Remedies

Acetaminophen (Tylenol)　Two tablets or caplets (650 mg) taken every four to six hours is the dose recommended on the label for pain from minor injuries, headache, or fever. Do not exceed the recommended dose unless specifically advised to do so by your clinician.

HERBAL REMEDIES

Capsaicin Cream　The cream made with the active ingredient found in chili peppers, capsaicin works by stimulating nerve sensors for pain in the area the cream is applied. The idea is that the pain threshold of the area treated is overwhelmed by this process, making the pain-sensing nerves in the treated area less sensitive to pain stimuli. The cream can cause a burning sensation, so keep it away from your eyes and wash your hands thoroughly after using. When applying, you may wish to use gloves to protect the skin on your hands. Different people have different reactions to capsaicin. To avoid the unpleasant burning sensation on the surface of the skin, you can numb the area you will treat with a benzocaine preparation (commonly found in teething creams). The numbing cream only affects the surface of the skin, so the capsaicin cream should still be effective on the underlying nerve pain. After applying the numbing cream, wait five to ten minutes before you rub on the capsaicin cream. Do not use capsaicin cream on surgical scars that are less than six months old or take capsaicin internally. Do not apply capsaicin cream on broken skin or wounds. Capsaicin cream may be used up to three to four times a day. To wash off capsaicin cream, use a little white vinegar.

> *When lifting objects, even if they are not heavy, be sure to use proper lifting technique. Bend your knees, don't just bend forward from the waist. Hold the object close to your body as you stand up. Better yet, don't lift heavy objects; ask for help.*

> *If you find capsaicin cream too irritating, remove it immediately with white vinegar rather than water.*

HOMEOPATHY

Arnica Cream   This homeopathic cream can be rubbed on sore areas. The skin must be intact, with no cuts or wounds (again, do not rub on tumor or on biopsy scars). Homeopathic arnica pills can also be taken internally. Try a 30x strength, taking four tablets as soon as possible after the injury, then four tablets every two to four hours for the next few days. Never take full-strength arnica internally, as it is not safe.

MASSAGE

Try massage, but ask the massage therapist to avoid massaging the tumor area.

Ice For an acute pain or injury, remember the acronym RICE (rest, ice, compression, elevation). Ice immediately applied after a strain or pull (within an hour or so) can prevent further swelling. Don't put ice directly on the injury. Wrap an ice pack or a bag of frozen peas with a towel (even a dish cloth will do) and then place the towel on the injury. Elevate the strained or pulled area of your body. This helps to drain fluid that can accumulate in the injured area and cause swelling. You can wrap an Ace bandage around the ice pack to keep pressure on the injured area. Another icing trick is to add a little rubbing alcohol (isopropyl) to a self-sealing bag of water and keep the mixture in your freezer for quick use. This fluid mixture never entirely freezes and molds beautifully over the body part you are icing.

> *Do not use ice before you exercise. Before activity, always use heat. Remember the phrase "warm up." Do not apply heat to skin areas within radiation treatment fields while you are on treatment.*

Use ice for fifteen-minute sessions every two hours for the first day or two after a strain or pull. Once the pain and swelling start to subside, you can apply heat. If the heat doesn't feel good, continue to use the ice for a day or two more.

VITAMINS AND MINERALS

Calcium and Magnesium Calcium and magnesium act as muscle relaxants. There are combination preparations, but to absorb any of the magnesium you need to take each mineral about two hours apart from the other for better absorption. Do not take magnesium with calcium-rich foods either. If you have multiple myeloma or breast or lung cancer, ask your clinician before adding supplemental calcium.

> *There are many different calcium salts. Calcium citrate has the best absorption.*

Potassium Bananas, avocados, citrus fruits, yogurt, spinach, and raisins all contain potassium. Potassium can also be found in nuts (almonds, cashews, and walnuts), molasses, lentils, sardines, and whole grain cereals. Do not take supplemental potassium unless advised to do so by your clinician.

USE WITH CARE

Aspirin   The recommended dose is two tablets (650 mg) every six hours. Always take aspirin with food.

NSAIDs   Nonsteroidal anti-inflammatories (NSAIDs) and aspirin can cause gastrointestinal bleeding and interfere with clotting. Do not take NSAIDs or aspirin if you have low red blood cell counts or low platelet counts (see *Bleeding and Bruising*, p. 61). On the other hand, NSAIDs are wonderful pain relievers for mild muscle and joint aches. NSAIDs are often used in pain management, but you may need some supervision because of your treatment. Follow the instructions on the label unless you are specifically advised otherwise by your clinician. Always take NSAIDs with food.

At the time of this writing, there are two versions of a newly approved nonsteroidal pain medication called a COX 2 inhibitor: celecoxib (Celebrex) and refecoxib (Vioxx). They are available only by prescription. These medications can be very helpful for aches and pains when you cannot use aspirin or other NSAIDs and when acetaminophen is not helpful. Ask your clinician about these new preparations to learn more.

The shorter acting NSAIDs such as ibuprofen (Advil, Nuprin, Motrin, etc.) are often recommended over the long-acting NSAIDs (naproxen, ketorelac, etc.) because it takes longer for the long-acting NSAIDs to clear from your system if you have a problem. Stick to ibuprofen if you are going to try an NSAID, or speak to your clinician first.

If a new ache or pain does not change after a day or two of rest and your choice of remedy, call your clinician.

WE DO NOT RECOMMEND

Do not ignore your aches and pains. They do not come with the territory just because you have a cancer diagnosis.

For more information on the complementary remedies discussed in this section, see chapter 3.

ANEMIA

Anemia is the term for a lower than normal red blood cell count and/or volume of red blood cells. The red blood cells (erythrocytes) serve a variety of important functions—but primarily they carry iron and supply oxygen throughout the body and help with the removal of carbon dioxide. These cells live longer than any of the other cells in the blood, approximately ninety to one hundred twenty days. The signs of anemia are what people often call "tired blood."

Signs of Anemia

The symptoms of fatigue and anemia can be easily confused. In fact, it is possible to suffer from both conditions at the same time. If you have a very low red cell count, you will probably feel tired much of the time, in addition to having one or more of the following symptoms:

- Shortness of breath—difficulty breathing while doing your normal daily activities. You may have trouble catching your breath when speaking or feel a heaviness in your chest.
- Dizziness with relatively slow movements (such as getting up out of bed or moving from sitting to standing).
- Paler skin than usual, including the pink tissue inside your mouth. Your lips may be bluish, or you may have pale creases on your palms (with darker skin, look for the pale color inside the mouth and what people sometimes describe as an ashiness in skin tone).

Call your clinician immediately if you have:

- Shortness of breath while lying down doing nothing
- Heart palpitations (a fast heartbeat with fast, shallow breathing) and/or chest pain or pressure
- Trouble breathing when you are not really doing anything (if just trying to say a complete sentence leaves you gasping for air)

Hematocrit and Hemoglobin

The lab test value called hematocrit is a measurement of the percentage of cells in your blood sample that are red blood cells. An estimate of the actual oxygen-carrying capacity is called hemoglobin. Mild anemia is a common side effect of cancer treatment over time. Blood test results can vary from lab to lab, so your results should always include the lab's normal value range of that test for comparison. The best treatment for anemia caused by cancer treatment is a blood transfusion, but this is done only when your hemoglobin and hematocrit levels are very low or you are experiencing the symptoms of low red blood cell counts (see below). Usually, your bone marrow is able to overcome the temporary low count; it just takes time for levels to return to normal. Since blood transfusions have their own risks, the benefit of waiting for recovery can often outweigh the risk of the transfusion. We recommend you get your clinician's opinion regarding at what point a transfusion could be necessary for you.

Diagnosis and Treatment Considerations

FACTORS THAT LEAD TO ANEMIA

- Chemotherapy treatment—can interfere with bone marrow production and kidney function, resulting in anemia (see more below)
- Poor diet—that is, not enough iron, vitamin B_{12}, folic acid, vitamin C, cobalt, copper, or essential amino acids
- Surgery to the stomach or upper intestine—can cause intestinal absorption problems
- Pregnancy
- Kidney disease
- Age (over forty)—some people begin to have trouble absorbing vitamin B_{12} from the diet, and this can lead to anemia. In this instance, if your blood test shows low levels of B_{12}, monthly injections of B_{12} are often prescribed.
- Bleeding—loss of blood from menstruation combined with a poor diet can lead to anemia. This is common in adolescent girls and young active women.
- Alcohol abuse—alcohol interferes with the absorption of nutrients needed for red blood cell formation.

BLEEDING

Bleeding is more likely to be the cause of your anemia when your symptoms are sudden. Bleeding can be internal, or blood can come out externally via your stool, vomit, urine, or nosebleeds that won't quit. If you notice large amounts of bright red blood in any body product, or black tarry-looking stools, call your clinician immediately.

DEHYDRATION

Dehydration can make your lab results appear better than they are because your blood becomes concentrated from lack of fluid. Don't ignore your physical symptoms, even if your lab results look fine.

PERNICIOUS ANEMIA

Pernicious anemia happens when your body does not store or absorb vitamin B_{12} from food adequately. This type of anemia can affect strict vegetarians who do not supplement their diet with B_{12} (which is found primarily in eggs, milk, and meat). Pernicious anemia is also a problem for older adults, who don't absorb B_{12} as well. As you age, your stomach stops secreting intrinsic factor, which is necessary for absorbing B_{12} from food. People who have had stomach or upper bowel surgery can also have difficulty with B_{12} absorption. Persistent tingling and numbness in the fingers and toes is usually the first symptom of pernicious anemia. A simple blood test can confirm this diagnosis. In strict vegetarians, pernicious anemia is prevented by adding B_{12} in the diet or supplementing with B_{12} vitamins. If you can't absorb B_{12} through diet or supplements, a monthly injection of B_{12} is recommended (this is usually recommended for those over forty). If you have had stomach or upper bowel surgery, a monthly injection of B_{12} is often required for the rest of your life. Strict vegetarians and vegans are advised to supplement their daily diet with 100 micrograms of oral B_{12}. To prevent stomach irritation, B_{12} should be taken with food and a full glass of liquid. If you are deficient in B_{12}, we advise you to consult your clinician for appropriate treatment.

SPLEEN

Very rarely, anemia can be related to a dysfunctional or hyperfunctional spleen. This diagnosis requires a number of tests to rule out all the usual possible causes of anemia before the spleen is suspected. This is sometimes a problem for people with non-Hodgkin's lymphoma.

CHEMOTHERAPY AND RADIATION

Chemotherapy and radiation affect red blood cells, but the effects are not usually seen until one to three months after the first treatment. This is because red blood cells live and work in your bloodstream for approximately 120 days, and treatment disrupts the replacement cells forming in the bone marrow, not the cells already out in your blood.

Anemia is a frequent side effect of cancer treatment because of the effects of radiation and chemotherapy on bone marrow. Your red blood cell count can also be affected by changes in diet and kidney function. Remember that radiation effects are dose related and will only have an effect on bone marrow if a large area of marrow-producing bone is in the field (for example, humerus [upper arm], pelvis, femur [thigh bone], spine, sternum, or ribs). Remember, radiation by itself does not usually affect the bone marrow significantly unless you have had chemotherapy before or during the radiation.

Prevention

LIFESTYLE MODIFICATIONS

If you suffer from diet-related anemia, we suggest working on your diet and increasing your intake of iron-containing foods. Iron is best absorbed through the foods you eat. Foods high in iron content are whole grains, lentils, beans (lima, navy, or butter), prune juice, nuts, leafy vegetables (except spinach and beet greens because of the presence of oxalic acid which impedes iron absorption), nettles, seaweed, liver, lean red meat, chicken, brewer's yeast, wheat germ, and fortified cereal. You can also get tiny amounts of iron from other dark green vegetables like romaine lettuce or lamb's quarters (a salad green). So if you love salad, use romaine lettuce in place of iceberg lettuce and add some toasted wheat germ for extra iron. Calcium absorption can interfere with iron absorption, so avoid eating calcium-rich foods within an hour of eating iron-rich foods. See *Appetite Problems*, p. 57, *Nutrition*, p. 244, and *Weight Loss and Gain*, p. 213, for more information on diet supplementation.

> *You absorb dietary iron better when it is taken in conjunction with vitamin C, so add citrus juices to your meals.*

> *You always want to prevent falling, so when you change positions, for example, from lying to sitting or sitting to standing, do it carefully. If you find you are dizzy regardless of your position, call your clinician.*

TAKE IT EASY

When you have low hemoglobin or low hematocrit levels, take it easy. It is a good idea to schedule important activities in the morning before you are tired and to avoid strenuous activities.

Remedies

CONVENTIONAL REMEDIES

Epoetin Alpha (Epogen, Procrit) This prescription drug stimulates a chemical response in your kidneys to tell the bone marrow to produce more red blood cells. This medication is given by injection, one to three times a week. It takes six to eight weeks before you find out if it is helpful or not. If there is no improvement after eight weeks, the manufacturer advises stopping the injections. This medication may be most helpful if you have a history of kidney failure or if you are taking chemotherapy that can affect the kidney function, for example, cisplatin or carboplatin.

HERBAL REMEDIES

Gentian If your anemia is a result of a poor appetite, you might want to try gentian, an herb used in mixers such as angostura bitters. It is known for improving digestion and stimulating the appetite. Gentian can be prepared as tea or taken as an extract. It is not recommended for people with hypertension (high blood pressure). Gentian can be found in tea or tincture (liquid) form. Do not take gentian if you suffer from ulcers or hypertension.

TRANSFUSION

A transfusion of red blood cells can help rescue red blood counts when they get too low. Your clinician will determine the need for transfusion on the basis of your symptoms and your hemoglobin and hematocrit results. Remember that transfusions are only a temporary fix for your low red blood cell count; they are not a cure.

USE WITH CARE

Folic Acid (Vitamin B9) and Folate Many people take folic acid as part of their daily vitamin supplements. However, if you are getting methotrexate or leucovorin, discuss supplementation of folic acid with your cancer clinician before you start treatment, as folic acid can interfere with these chemotherapies' effectiveness. Supplemental folic acid is also not recommended if you have been diagnosed with pernicious anemia (see *Anemia*, p 40.)

IRON

Do not take iron as a dietary supplement unless it is specifically recommended to you by your clinician. Supplemental iron is not an appropriate treatment by itself for severe anemia. Severe anemia may need to be treated with intravenous iron or a blood transfusion, depending on the cause. If you do take supplemental iron, remember to take it on an empty stomach (at least one hour before or two hours after eating or drinking anything). Do not take iron supplements with other medications. Iron often causes stomach upset and constipation (see *Constipation*, p. 88). Also keep in mind that iron is poorly absorbed as a supplement when combined with anything other than citrus juice. If you are taking supplemental iron, it will usually take a few months to see an improvement in your blood counts.

WE DO NOT RECOMMEND

Alcohol   Cut back on alcohol consumption. Alcohol interferes with nutrient absorption.

Spinach   Sadly, your mother and Popeye were wrong on this subject. Spinach would be a wonderful source of iron except for the fact that it has another chemical component (oxalic acid) that prevents you from being able to absorb the iron from it. Eat spinach because you like it but not for its iron content. The same is true for beet greens.

For more information on the complementary remedies discussed in this section, see chapter 3.

ANGER

People diagnosed with cancer often feel angry. It is completely understandable to feel this way. It isn't fair that you got this disease. In fact, there is no fair disease.

There are other anger-producing aspects of cancer treatment. Dealing with the healthcare establishment, with insurance and other financial considerations, can cause frustration and anger. Having to disrupt your life and routines for treatment can cause anger. Not feeling in control of your life can cause anger. You may even feel angry with yourself for things you have done that you believe may have led to your cancer. You may find yourself angry or short-tempered with friends and family.

Anger is a very powerful motivator that can be used positively or negatively. Anger can give you strength to take action if you turn it around. It can help you to focus on your needs and be more assertive about getting those needs met. However, anger will be destructive if it prevents you from taking care of yourself or if it isolates you from those around you. If anger is not expressed and is turned inward, it can lead to depression.

Diagnosis and Treatment Considerations

While there are many aspects of cancer treatment itself that can cause anger and frustration, anger can also be a side effect of medication. Atropine, used for intense diarrhea, and scopalamine, used for motion sickness and nausea, are examples of common medications that can have the side effect of feeling "hot, dry, and mad." The adrenocorticoids (cortisone, hydrocortisone, dexamethasone, methyl prednisone, methyl prednisolone, prednisone, prednisilone) are also famous for changing the way you feel. Some people feel very edgy and tense while taking one of these for more than a day or two. Almost any medication that regulates heart function, blood pressure, or mood has the potential to make you feel angry. If you suspect your medication may be causing this side effect, discuss your suspicion with the clinician who prescribed the medication and find out if the dose or medication can be changed.

If a particular medication is not the cause of your problem, or if the medication has triggered emotions you've been trying to avoid, try to figure out what or whom you are really angry at. Does this anger originate from experiences you had in the past? Are you angry with specific people in your life? If there are people you need to forgive, now is a good time to work on it. You may need to let go of the angry feelings and move on. Right now, you can't afford to waste any of your energy on past resentments. You need all your strength for healing (see *Stress*, p. 264).

Remedies

AROMATHERAPY

Rose Oil and Lavender Oil   Do you ever wonder why roses are the flowers of choice after couples have fights? It is because the scent of roses has traditionally been thought to alleviate anger. Lavender is another soothing aroma. Try putting five drops of rose oil or lavender oil into a warm bath. You can also inhale the fragrance directly from the bottle or put a few drops into a diffuser.

BACH FLOWER REMEDIES

Specific remedies are used to treat specific manifestations of anger.

Pine—if you are angry at yourself
Willow—for dealing with a circumstance you feel is unfair
Gentian—used for feelings of anger and frustration

COMMUNICATION

Anger can sometimes be a mask for other feelings, such as sadness or fear. Talking to someone about your feelings can help sort out your emotions and begin to give you a sense of control over what is happening to you. As with every other emotion, it is a good idea to fully experience your anger and then move on. This means that instead of rising above it or putting on a happy face, tell someone how angry you feel. Try it. You may be surprised at how relieved you feel after you finally say the words.

HOMEOPATHY

Take the homeopathic remedy that applies to your situation one to three times a day over a two-day period. We recommend you stop using the remedy as soon as symptoms go away.

Natrum mur—for people who hold grudges and feel betrayed
Staphysagrai—for strong emotions of anger that have been suppressed
Nux vomica—for feelings of impatience and irritability

MEDITATION, RELAXATION, AND YOGA

Meditation and relaxation techniques can be wonderful tools to help you deal with anger. These practices help you to let go of emotions that are not useful to you by focusing your energy and attention on the present moment. Yoga poses are a good way to calm strong emotions, and yoga breathing practices are especially helpful. See *Meditation,* p. 242, and *Relaxation,* p. 252, for more information on exercises you can try.

VITAMINS AND MINERALS

It is sometimes difficult to pay attention to healthy eating when you are receiving cancer treatment. However, nutrition is very important at this time.

Calcium and Magnesium The minerals calcium and magnesium can have a calming effect on mood. If you can't get enough calcium and magnesium through food, you can take a supplement, but be aware that calcium and magnesium supplements are not appropriate for everyone (see below).

  Calcium can be found in foods such as cheese, yogurt, salmon, broccoli, and almonds. Calcium supplements are not recommended for those at risk of hypercalcemia (for example, if you have metastatic breast cancer, some lung cancers, or multiple myeloma); it is a good idea to speak to your clinician before adding calcium supplements to your diet.

  Magnesium can also be found in nuts, seafood, bananas, and wheat germ. Magnesium is absorbed best when taken at least an hour before or two hours after eating calcium-rich food or taking a calcium supplement. Additional magnesium supplementation is not recommended for those with renal failure or diarrhea.

For more information on the complementary remedies discussed in this section, see chapter 3.

ANXIETY

Your heart races, your breathing quickens, your palms sweat. You may feel restless and jittery, as if you are in danger. This physical reaction, known as the "fight or flight" response, is a basic survival instinct. It prepares you physically and mentally to confront danger or to run for your life. This mechanism served our ancestors well when they had to survive the threats of wild animals and unexpected danger on a daily basis. In modern life, however, constantly experiencing this rush of hormones in response to everyday problems only makes you feel more anxious.

Living with a diagnosis of cancer is stressful. Waiting for the results of tests is stressful. Undergoing medical procedures is stressful. Worrying about the future is stressful. Just hearing the word *cancer* itself can produce tremendous anxiety. Acknowledging your anxiety is the first step toward dealing with it.

Diagnosis and Treatment Considerations

BRAIN METASTASES

Very rarely, anxiety can also be a result of brain metastases. No one knows exactly why this happens, but it is possible that when brain metastases are in an area that controls physical comfort, breathing, or circulation, the effect can be anxiety. Brain metastases are often treated with radiation to stop both the symptoms and the discomfort.

BREATHING

A common cause of anxiety is not breathing effectively. There are various conditions that can affect your body's ability to get and use oxygen, including lung cancer, lung metastases, pain, congestive heart failure, a lung infection, a blood clot in the lungs, an allergic reaction, fatigue, or severe weakness. The more mundane causes of not breathing well can be wearing too tight a belt around the waist, slouching, severe nasal congestion, and physical tension in your shoulder, neck, or chest muscles. The best way to control anxiety related to one of these conditions is to treat the underlying cause. If the underlying cause of your breathing problem cannot be changed, it is helpful to be vigilant with deep breathing exercises and to move about a little more slowly so that fast, shallow breathing is not triggered. If certain activities make you anxious, stop the activity for a moment and catch your breath. This often can make the feeling of anxiety disappear (see *Breathing Problems*, p. 67).

MEDICATIONS

Some medications can cause anxiety as a side effect. After discussing with your clinician the possibility that a medication is the cause of your anxiety problem, it is entirely reasonable to stop or change a medication. Here are some of the most common offenders.

Adrenocorticoids (Cortisone, Hydrocortisone, Dexamethasone, Methyl Prednisone, Methyl Prednisolone, Prednisone, Prednisilone)   These medications mimic your body's own steroid, adrenaline, the hormone your body secretes to help you to flee when you feel anxious. Be advised that adrenocorticoids cannot just be stopped suddenly but must be tapered off with the help of your clinician.

Albuterol (Proventil) Inhalers   These are beta 2 selective adrenergic agonist bronchodilators used in the treatment of asthma, emphysema (chronic obstructive pulmonary disease, or COPD), and other breathing problems. This class of medication can increase your heart rate slightly when used in an inhaler for bronchodilation. Anxiety is more likely to be a problem with higher doses of inhaled albuterol.

Antihistamines and Decongestants   Anxiety is a side effect of caffeine and ephedrine, which are ingredients in many common antihistamines, decongestants, and cold/flu remedies, especially those formulated to prevent drowsiness. You may need to try different products to find one that doesn't make you feel anxious.

Chlorpromazine Hydrochloride (Thorazine)   Thorazine is often used for problems with intractable hiccups (see *Hiccups,* p. 143). It is chemically similar to prochlorperazine (Compazine; see below) and can cause a similar adverse side effect of anxiety. The same guidelines apply for this drug as to prochlorperazine.

Prochlorperazine (Compazine)   This excellent antinausea (and sometimes antianxiety) medication has a rare adverse side effect of causing anxiety in some people. If you notice that your anxiety started or significantly increased with the use of prochlorperazine, tell your clinician and ask for a different antinausea medication.

Opioid Pain Medication   People have different side effects when taking different opioids. If you suspect that your anxiety coincides with either a new medication or a higher dose of a pain medication, you need to discuss this with the clinician who prescribed the opioid. Most side effects with opioids go away after three days or so of use. If this is not true for you, you may need to try a different opioid, or a combination of medications tailored for your particular situation, to minimize intolerable side effects.

   If you have recently lowered your dose of opioid and experience anxiety, it may be related to weaning off the opioid dose too quickly.

This is often alleviated when the clinician helps to lower the opioid dose more slowly. Your withdrawal symptoms are not a problem of addiction but simply of decreasing your medication dose too quickly.

Prevention

If your anxiety is not related to medication or breathing difficulties, you will need to find the source of your anxiety so you can deal with it. Asking yourself questions about your anxiety can be helpful. Have you experienced panic attacks or treatment for anxiety in the past? What worked then? If you were in therapy or took medication and it was helpful, try it again. Don't be embarrassed to ask for help. Anxiety is an experience that many people suffer through even though it can be successfully treated.

Don't ever let anxiety stop you from getting your treatment or procedures. You are too important to neglect your care.

Maybe you are anxious because you have specific fears that you are not telling anyone about. Increasing your understanding of your disease is a simple way to diffuse the fears related to tests and treatments. Don't be afraid to talk to your clinicians. Ask as many questions as you need to allay your anxiety. Your clinicians can ease your mind about some of your fears about treatment, or they may be able to prescribe an antianxiety medication that can help you through this difficult period (see below). Some people are reluctant to take medications for anxiety; however, these medications can be very effective to help you get some control back and can be tapered off when you start to feel better and no longer need them.

Remedies

AROMATHERAPY

Try the essential oils lavender, ylang-ylang, or marjoram. Add six drops of one of these essential oils to a hot bath or a diffuser.

BACH FLOWER REMEDIES

Rescue Remedy—a mix of five flower essences, this is the classic remedy for an anxiety attack. You can carry a small bottle of Rescue Remedy with you and put a few drops under your tongue whenever you start feeling anxious.

Aspen—for ongoing feelings of foreboding.

Red chestnut—if you constantly worry about other people.

BATHS

A neutral bath (slightly less than body temperature, which is around 96 degrees) can relieve feelings of anxiety. You can check the temperature with a regular thermometer. Stay in the bath for twenty minutes or for as long as is comfortable, adding more water as needed. This is not recommended if you are neutropenic or have low hemoglobin or hematocrit (anemia).

BREATHING EXERCISES

One of the most effective ways to manage anxiety is always with you: your breath. Anxiety is your body's effort to be ready for anything. The anticipation response starts with breathing quickly in short, shallow breaths. Breathing this way will quickly cause you to hyperventilate, increasing your sense of anxiety. Do you remember the famous photographs of girls waiting for the Beatles or Elvis Presley to arrive at airports? Many of the girls were fainting. Remember the remedy? It was breathing with a paper bag over the mouth and nose. Breathing into a paper bag will prevent hyperventilation by forcing deeper inhalations, thereby allowing your lungs to function more thoroughly. Don't use a plastic bag, as this is a suffocation device. The other benefit of deep, slow breathing is that it is very difficult to feel anxious at the same time that you are breathing in slowly and deeply. You can simulate a paper bag by cupping your hands together over your mouth and nose, closing your eyes, and focusing on your breath. Or, with your mouth closed, breathe with one nostril, closing the other nostril with your finger. Try it right now for a few minutes to see how it feels. You should feel an immediate sensation of calm. Remember this technique to use whenever you are feeling anxious.

A Simple Breathing Exercise

Close your eyes.

Try to sit up straight or lie flat.

Make sure your back is well supported.
Focus only on your breathing.
Breathe
Slowly
In and out
Through your nose.
Let any thoughts that come into your mind drift away like clouds.

The beauty of breathing exercises is that you can do them anywhere and at any time. Of course, keep your eyes open if you need to be aware of your surroundings or if you are driving. If you practice breathing exercises, you will find that you will even be able to do them without having to close your eyes.

COMMUNICATION

Talk to people around you. Share your feelings with your clinicians, your friends, and your family. Join a support group and talk to people experiencing similar issues. Many cancer centers and cancer organizations have programs where you can be connected with someone who has experienced a similar diagnosis and treatment plan. This one-to-one contact can be invaluable as a reality check and support system. Or talk to a trained cancer counselor. If you keep your feelings to yourself, you may become more anxious. The organization Cancercare (www.cancercare.org) has compiled a list of various support groups, including online support groups and phone support groups.

> *If you have trouble sleeping because your mind races, try to learn a relaxation technique.* See Relaxation, *p. 252,* Meditation, *p. 242,* Sleep Problems, *p. 192.*

CONVENTIONAL MEDICATIONS

Antianxiety medications provide an excellent way to quickly cope with anxiety symptoms. There are quite a few antianxiety medications; we only discuss here the ones commonly used for anxiety control during cancer treatment. Many medications known to help relieve anxiety also help in other symptom management. For instance, prochlorperazine (Compazine) can be used as an antianxiety agent, but in cancer care it is more often used for controlling nausea. Do not combine conventional antianxiety medications with any herbal antianxiety remedies.

Benzodiazepines: Lorazepam (Ativan) and Alprazolam (Xanax)   The benzodiazepine lorazepam is a wonderful antianxiety medication because of its quick action and effectiveness. Lorazepam comes in an oral version that can be taken by letting it dissolve under the tongue or swallowing. It usually starts to work within five to fifteen minutes. This sublingual version is especially helpful when you feel nauseated. Lorazepam starts to work quickly and the oral version lasts about four to six hours. Beware that lorazepam can interfere with your dreaming and the quality of your sleep. With some people, there is a rare adverse side effect of agitation, making lorazepam an inappropriate medication for them. Alprazolam works similarly to lorazepam although it is slightly longer acting.

EXERCISE

Take a brisk fifteen-minute walk. You'll be surprised how much calmer you will feel.

HERBAL REMEDIES

It is important not to combine antianxiety remedies, whether conventional or complementary. More is not better, or safe. For mild anxiety, herbal remedies can be very helpful. With more severe, debilitating anxiety, conventional remedies are recommended.

Chamomile   Chamomile tea has a known calming effect, especially when used before bedtime. We do not recommend drinking more than three cups of chamomile tea a day. Do not add honey if you are neutropenic (see *Neutropenia*, p. 178). If you are allergic to chrysanthemums, daisies, ragweed, or yarrow, we don't recommend using chamomile, as it may cause a similar allergic reaction.

Hops   Usually thought of as an ingredient in the making of beer, hops has also been used for many years in Europe as a treatment for insomnia and nervousness. When you are having trouble sleeping, try taking two capsules of a freeze-dried extract of hops before you go to sleep or drink a cup of hops tea before bedtime.

Kava Kava   Found in the Polynesian islands, kava kava (Piper methysticum) has been used for more than three thousand years as a calming remedy. The active ingredients in kava kava, called kava lactones, have a sedative effect. In a recent clinical study of anxiety in Germany, kava did as well as tricyclic antidepressants such as amytriptyline (Elavil) and benzodiazepines such as lorazepam and oxazepam. The advantage of kava kava was that it remedied anxiety without the problems of tolerance that built up over time with either of the prescription medications. It is suggested that you take this herb for no more than three months at a time. We do not recommend using kava kava if you have Parkinson's disease.

Passionflower   This herb (Passiflora incarnata) acts as a mild tranquilizer and can help you get to sleep. You can buy it in tea, tincture, or extract form. Although the exact mechanism of its action is unclear, the German Commission E has found it to be helpful for insomnia. Try a soothing cup of passionflower tea before bedtime.

Valerian   An herbal sedative, valerian has been shown to be an effective remedy for anxiety and insomnia. Some people find that valerian has a strange odor. You can take valerian as a tea, as a tincture (liquid) extract, or in capsules of the freeze-dried extract. It is usually recommended in the tincture (liquid) form. A few people are sensitive to valerian, and they may find that the recommended dose leaves them with a feeling like a hangover. If this is the case, cut back the dose or try a different remedy altogether. As valerian works like any other sedative, it is very important that you don't combine it with other sleeping pills, antianxiety medications, or alcohol. Be patient; valerian may take two to four weeks to become effective.

> *As these herbs function as mild sedatives, do not combine kava kava or valerian with each other or any other sedative or tranquilizer, including alcohol.*

HOMEOPATHY

For anxiety that relates to a specific event such as a treatment or a test, there are three homeopathic remedies that may be helpful. Try one for a day and see how you feel.

Gelsenium—for times when you feel anxious in a physical way (for example, physically weak in the knees)

Argentum nitricum—for strong nervous anticipation

Lycopodium—for people who suffer from a fear of failure or appearing foolish

MASSAGE

Massage is a wonderful way to relieve tension and anxiety. If you can afford a professional massage, this is a wonderful gift to give yourself. When you tense up emotionally, your muscles can tense up as well. We recommend you ask the massage therapist to avoid massaging an identified tumor site.

Simple Calming Self-massage Here is a simple massage you can give yourself easily. Take the palm of your hand and massage the solar plexus (the area just below your breastbone). Stroke gently in circular motions, concentrating on the movement and how it feels in your body. Try this while you lie in bed or any time you feel anxious.

MUSIC

Music can have a wonderfully relaxing effect, especially music with a slow, steady beat. What relaxes you is very individual. Some people prefer slow, quiet music or classical music, while others like country or folk or nature sounds. A recent study of music's effect on cancer patients found that listening to music of the patient's choice helped alleviate the anxiety patients experienced when returning to the hospital or undergoing chemotherapy. Try making a special tape of music and sounds you find relaxing and reassuring to play whenever you start feeling tense or anxious.

NUTRITION

There are certain foods that reportedly have a calming effect, such as whole grains and oats. Diets heavy in potatoes and pasta have been used successfully to calm people with certain organic brain conditions not associated with cancer. "Comfort foods" are usually high in carbohydrates and can ease feelings of tension.

Alcohol Anxiety and depression are often related. Since alcohol is a depressant, try to avoid overindulging. A glass of wine now and again can be relaxing, but try not to use alcohol to self-medicate for anxiety.

For more information on the complementary remedies discussed in this section, see chapter 3.

APPETITE PROBLEMS

We all know the importance of eating and sharing meals. However, appetites can and do change while on any treatment, including cancer treatment. If you are having trouble eating, let your loved ones know this is an effect of being under treatment. Although they may feel they are helping you by encouraging you to eat, it's important to let them know what your appetite is like and what would be helpful for you to eat.

Questions To Ask Yourself

- How is your appetite? Is it increasing or decreasing?
- Are you experiencing changes in food tastes (see *Taste Changes*, p. 204) or a lessening of desire to eat?
- Are you experiencing difficulty with the act of eating? (See *Breathing Problems*, p. 67, *Cough*, p. 94, *Depression*, p. 102, *Infection*, p. 151, *Mouth Sores*, p. 159, *Nasal Congestion*, p. 168, *Weight Loss or Gain*, p. 213.)
- Is your nausea from chemotherapy or abdominal radiation under control? (See *Nausea and Vomiting*, p. 170.)

If you don't feel well, you're probably not going to have a big appetite. However, if you are losing one-half to one pound a week, refer to *Weight Loss and Gain*, p. 213, *Taste Changes*, p. 204, or *Nutrition*, p. 244. If you are losing one or more pounds a week, you need to call your clinician. Usually the goal while on cancer therapy is to maintain your weight unless recommended otherwise by your clinician.

> *Refer to* Nutrition, *p. 244, after reading this section for tips on other ways to improve your diet.*

Diagnosis and Treatment Considerations

Most cancers and cancer treatments affect appetite in one way or another. The reasons for this problem can run the gamut from mechanical changes as a result of surgery to a purely psychological reaction such as a negative association with food that prevents you from eating well.

MEDICATIONS THAT CAN INCREASE APPETITE

- Adrenocorticoids (cortisone, hydrocortisone, dexamethasone, methyl prednisone, methyl prednisolone, prednisone, prednisilone)
- Megestrol (Megace)
- THC (Marinol)—the active ingredient in marijuana
- Common breast cancer chemotherapy regimens

MEDICATIONS THAT DECREASE APPETITE

Most chemotherapies, biological response modifiers, and sedating medications can have an effect on your appetite. In fact, any medication that causes fatigue, sedation, queasiness, or heartburn can cause a decrease in appetite.

OTHER CAUSES OF DECREASE IN APPETITE

Anytime your gastrointestinal system is affected by treatment, you can notice a change in your appetite. This is true regardless of whether the treatment was chemotherapy, surgery, or radiation. Be aware that depression can also cause a lack of appetite (see *Depression*, p. 102).

Your diet itself can cause a decrease in appetite if you are on a therapy that involves a special diet. You may also wish to refer to *Nutrition*, p. 244, after reading this section, for tips on how to load up your snacks and improve your nutrition.

Prevention

If your appetite is poor, drink more fluids with calories and nutrients rather than plain water. We recommend drinking creamed soups, shakes, and frappes, so you get fluid and food all in one. Ask your clinician if it is all right for you to have a glass of wine before meals. Alcohol is a mild appetite stimulant. (Remember how good those pretzels and chips look when you're drinking a beer?) Or drink a little lemonade to stimulate appetite half an hour before eating.

What to do if you have too much appetite:

- Stay away from high-calorie snacks.
- Stay away from no-fat foods, as well, since you'll probably end up eating more calories just trying to satisfy your appetite.
- Go for a walk after you eat.
- Don't beat yourself up for the weight gain. Know that it's a result of the medication and not a lack of willpower.
- See *Weight Loss and Gain*, p. 213.

What to do to increase your appetite:

- Eat only foods that appeal to you.
- Forget only three meals a day. Eat when you feel like it, nibble when you don't feel up to a whole meal. Just keep eating.
- Try fruit smoothies made with yogurt or a soy-based product so that you have something to sip on throughout the day.
- Try to arrange to eat meals with someone.
- Soup is an excellent way to get fluid, calories, and nutrients in one clever package.
- Vary what you eat to prevent food boredom.

Remedies

AROMATHERAPY

Certain fragrances increase appetite. Try *black pepper, orange,* or *ginger oil.* You can inhale these oils or put a few drops into a bath or in an aromatherapy diffuser.

EXERCISE

Increase your activities as much as you are able. If you have the energy, take a short walk half an hour before eating.

HERBAL REMEDIES

Anise (Fennel)   A mild appetite stimulant, anise can be eaten as a vegetable, prepared as a tea, or used as a condiment.

Cumin   A condiment used in curries, cumin is also a mild appetite stimulant.

Dandelion   This herb has been used for medicinal purposes for hundreds of years. One use of dandelion is as a mild appetite stimulant. Try dandelion tea, dandelion wine, or dandelion as salad greens. Fresh dandelion is only available in the early spring. Do not use if dehydrated.

Gentian   An herb used in alcohol preparations such as angostura bitters, gentian is reported to improve digestion. Gentian can be prepared as tea or taken as an extract. Gentian is not advised for those with hypertension (high blood pressure) or ulcers.

Ginger   This herb stimulates appetite by helping peristalsis. You can take ginger in many different forms. Try ginger tea, candied ginger root, fresh or pickled ginger, or Jamaican-style ginger beer. American ginger ale is usually not strong enough in the ginger department, even though it tastes good.

Milk Thistle (Silybum Marianum)   A liver protective herb, milk thistle is also used as a remedy for appetite loss. Take this herb in pill or extract, as it is not effective as a tea. Do not use if in treatment for hepatocellular cancer or liver metastases.

Parsley   Besides keeping your breath fresh, parsley aids in digestion. Do not use parsley oil (extract), as it is toxic.

RELAXATION

Relaxation exercises before eating help the appetite (see *Relaxation,* p. 252).

YOGA

Yoga is good for improving appetite. Try taking a yoga class or using a yoga tape at home.

USE WITH CARE

Marijuana or THC (Marinol)   Many people have heard that marijuana is effective for nausea prevention and as an aid to increasing appetite. We do not recommend smoking marijuana as there are definitely health risks to your lungs, esophagus, mouth, and heart related to smoking anything. However, the active ingredient of marijuana, THC, is now available by prescription in pill form, called Marinol.

This medication has been found to be more effective and better tolerated when the dose is started low and is slowly increased over a week or so to prevent what some people experience as an unpleasant sensation of euphoria. Speak to your clinician about whether THC is something that could help your appetite. THC is not recommended for the elderly as it can cause decreased cognition. Some people don't ever tolerate the euphorialike side effect, no matter how it is dosed, making this medication unhelpful for them.

WE DO NOT RECOMMEND

Licorice Root   Licorice is often used to stimulate the appetite. However, an ingredient in licorice root called glycrrhizin can be dangerous and overstimulating for your heart. It is also the ingredient that gives licorice its sweetness. You can, however, purchase licorice that has had that ingredient removed. This type of licorice, called deglycyrrhizinated licorice, or DGL, has been shown to be effective against heartburn and to soothe the digestive tract.

For more information on the complementary remedies discussed in this section, see chapter 3.

BLEEDING AND BRUISING

New unexplained bleeding is a symptom to take seriously. Bleeding for which there is no obvious source—other than a cut, a scratch, an irritated hemorrhoid, or too forceful a nose blow, is cause for concern. If you are taking an anticoagulant (blood thinner) such as heparin, warfarin (Coumadin), or aspirin, bleeding happens more easily but still needs to be taken seriously. If you have new bleeding or bruising that you can't explain or if you are concerned, call your clinician.

Various lab tests can be used by clinicians to keep an eye on what are called your bleed times and clotting functions. These tests include platelet count, PT and PTT (bleed times), and liver func-

Blood-thinning agents should not be combined with many medications. Be sure to inform your clinicians of all the medications you are taking, including over-the-counter products, vitamins, herbs, and supplements.

tion studies, among others. Other than the platelet count, which is usually done every time you have a complete blood test (CBC), these other tests are not done frequently unless there is a specific reason to monitor the results.

Diagnosis and Treatment Considerations

You could be prone to bruising or bleeding if:

- You have previously experienced a major bleed, such as gastrointestinal bleeding or a serious nosebleed that landed you in the emergency room
- You have had chemotherapy recently
- You have recently had several weeks of radiation to a marrow-producing bone (humerus [upper arm], sternum, spine, ribs, pelvis, femur [thigh])
- You have had a pronounced high fever
- You have engaged in strenuous exercise or other strenuous activity

CAUSES OF NEW BLEEDING AND/OR BRUISING

Platelets, the sticky building blocks of clotting, are related to blood cells. They have the same "grandparents" in the bone marrow and are therefore affected by the bone-marrow suppression caused by many cancer treatments. Aspirin, ibuprofen (and most other NSAIDs), and fevers all interfere with the effectiveness of platelets. In the normal life span of the platelet, it circulates in the bloodstream for about a week and is then taken out of service by the lymph system.

> *It is completely reasonable for a clinician to delay cancer treatment if you have a low platelet count—usually below one hundred thousand or so.*

MEDICATIONS THAT CAN CAUSE BLEEDING

Aspirin   A daily dose of aspirin is often recommended for older adults to prevent stroke and other serious vascular problems. However, the thinning effect aspirin has on the blood can compromise clotting and promote bleeding.

Cimetidine (Zantac), Estrogen Replacement Therapy, and Hydrochloroth-
   iazide (HCTZ)   These medications all can interfere with platelet
   function.

Warfarin (Coumadin)   If you have a central venous catheter or a history of clots, you may be prescribed an anticoagulant such as
   warfarin (Coumadin). The anticoagulants interfere with the coagulation process, making you generally more prone to bruising and
   bleeding.

WHEN YOU HAVE A BLOOD TEST

If you have low platelets (thrombocytopenia) or are on a blood-thinning
agent, you are likely to bruise every time you get a blood test. To help
with clotting and to prevent bruising after the needle is pulled out, be
sure to hold the cotton or gauze pad down tightly after the blood is
drawn. We recommend putting pressure on the puncture site (with your
thumb) for at least three to five minutes.

WHAT TO DO WHEN YOU HAVE LOW PLATELETS

If you fall or cut or scrape yourself, immediately apply pressure to the area.
For cuts and scrapes, apply pressure with whatever you are using to absorb
the blood such as a towel or gauze. Raise the injured part if possible, apply ice for ten minutes after removing the initial pressure, and then wash
the area gently with mild soap and water. When the bleeding has stopped,
if possible, leave the wounded area open to air for better healing. Don't
take aspirin or NSAIDs such as ibuprofen if you have a low platelet
count. Instead take acetaminophen or your prescribed medication for
pain (see *Aches and Pains,* p. 33).

   At the time of this writing, there are now two versions of an anti-
inflammatory called a COX 2 inhibitor, celecoxib (Celebrex) and rofe-
coxib (Vioxx). These medications are theoretically safe to take with
bleeding problems, but speak to your clinician first. They are by prescription only.

When To Call Your Clinician   When you have low platelets, you may
   notice bruises but not recall having bumped anything. If you notice
   a new purplish rash on your arms or legs but have no other rash side
   effects (itchiness, bumpiness), this could be petichiae, which are

minihemorrhagic spots. Petichiae are a symptom of inappropriate clotting in the capillaries and are often accompanied by fever. If you think you have petichiae, take your temperature and call your clinician immediately. It is possible that you may not be showing a fever yet, but the petichiae may be an early warning of one.

If you have low platelets and any of the following conditions, call your clinician immediately:

- Red or black blood in your stool
- Coughing up of red blood or what look like coffee grounds
- A nosebleed that won't stop
- Blood in your urine
- Taking a fall or twisting your elbow, shoulder, hip, knee, or ankle
- Bleeding anywhere that won't stop after a few minutes

Prevention

You should always try to prevent bruises and bleeding while on a treatment regimen. Follow these steps to prevent bleeding:

- If you take ibuprofen or other NSAIDs, always take them with food. Don't take NSAIDs if you have low platelets, are on warfarin (Coumadin) or heparin, or take daily aspirin without your clinician's supervision.
- Be sure to wear shoes when you are walking outside. Pay attention while walking. Look at the surface of the ground and at the objects you are walking around. Be careful not to fall.
- Try not to burn your mouth or tongue with hot liquids or foods.
- If your platelets are low, blow your nose gently.
- Don't pick your nose.
- Don't lift heavy objects. Get help to carry groceries, for example.
- Don't rub your eyes.

DENTAL CARE

Brush your teeth with the softest toothbrush you can buy (try a soft child's toothbrush). If you didn't floss your teeth before, don't begin while you are on treatment or if your clinician tells you that you have low platelets. Wait until you are finished with treatment to work on better gum care.

GROOMING

- When you wash, be gentle to your skin and thorough only in those areas that need it (hands, underarms, your privates).
- Use a mild soap for cleansing. We don't recommend any antibacterial or antiperspirant soaps.
- Rinse soap off your skin completely. Bar soaps rinse off more easily than liquid soaps (see *Infection*, p. 151, *Immunity*, p. 233).
- Cut your fingernails and toenails carefully with a clean clipper.
- Use an electric shaver if you have low platelets (under one hundred thousand) whether you are male or female.
- Don't use tampons when your platelets are under one hundred thousand.

SEX

Use an appropriate lubricant during sexual intercourse. There are specific water-based products for this use that are safe to use internally and on condoms. Do not use petroleum jelly or petrolatum (see *Sex and Sexuality*, p. 256). If your platelet count is below fifty thousand, sexual intercourse is not recommended.

IMPROVING PLATELET COUNTS

Because platelets have a life span of just under a week, a low platelet count usually starts to improve after a week or so if you are not on treatment. Research is being done to come up with a medication that is effective in stimulating platelet production. This medication would be similar to the medications used to stimulate white and red blood cells. As of this writing, one product is currently on the market, called oprelvekin (Neumega). If your platelets are severely depleted, you may be advised to have a platelet transfusion. If anyone you know has told you that he or she would like to help you, ask them to donate platelets or other blood products at their local hospital or blood bank. Blood products are always needed, especially platelets.

PETS

If your pet bites or scratches, do not play with it while you have low platelets. Keep your skin intact. A scratch from a pet can put you at risk for bleeding and infection.

WE DO NOT RECOMMEND

Herbs   It is probably not a good idea to use herbs to stop bleeding while on cancer treatment. Coagulation (clotting) is an extremely delicate process involving various chemicals in precise balance in the body. As cancer and cancer treatment affect these chemical balances, it is best to first treat the cancer or modify the cancer treatment, which will in turn, hopefully, get your bleeding process back under control.

> *As always, we recommend you select herbs from quality manufacturers, listen to advice from respected experts in the field (like Varro Tyler), and trust your body's own reactions. We believe it is always important to be mindful of possible interactions between all the medications you are taking, whether they are herbs, vitamins, or prescription drugs.*

Feverfew, Garlic, Ginger, and Ginkgo   These herbs interfere with platelet action; discontinue them if you are experiencing problems with bleeding or bruising. Never take any of these herbs in combination with prescribed blood thinners such as warfarin, heparin, or aspirin.

Ginseng   While some guides to drugs and herb interactions claim that ginseng affects the anticoagulant effects of warfarin (Coumadin), Varro Tyler refutes this in his monthly column (*Prevention,* January 2000). After his review of the studies involving ginseng and warfarin, he concludes that there was no interaction between ginseng and warfarin.

For more information on the complementary remedies discussed in this section, see chapter 3.

BREATHING PROBLEMS

Most of us breathe twenty-four hours a day without giving it a second thought. The only time you probably find yourself thinking about your breathing is when you are having a problem with it. We recommend that you give a thought to your breathing every so often, especially when you are not experiencing a problem, to appreciate your lungs' role in keeping your body chemically balanced and energized.

Shortness of Breath

If you have trouble catching your breath when you change position (from lying to sitting, or sitting to standing) or if you cannot complete a sentence without gasping, you should call your clinician (see *Anemia*, p. 40). If your shortness of breath is a chronic problem, below are tips on ways to manage your breathing better.

Diagnosis and Treatment Considerations

Chest surgery, lung cancer, and brain and lung metastases can affect your breathing. Breathing exercises are helpful in these situations to learn how to control your breathing and prevent hyperventilation. Pain can also affect breathing (see *Cancer Pain*, p. 69).

CHEMOTHERAPY AND BIOLOGICAL RESPONSE MODIFIERS

Some chemotherapies are known to interfere with breathing:

- Bleomycin—call your clinician immediately with sudden breathing problems
- Cyclophosphamide (Cytoxan)
- Doxorubicin (Adriamycin) and liposomal doxorubicin (Doxil)
- Etoposide (VP 16)
- Interleukin
- Interferon alpha (Roferon, Intron A)

If you experience changes in breathing while on these chemotherapies, let your clinician know.

Other health problems that can affect your breathing are:

- Asthma
- COPD (chronic obstructive pulmonary disease, or emphysema)
- Congestive heart failure
- Poorly controlled diabetes
- Abdominal swelling (ascites)

With these conditions, breathing problems can be more complicated to manage. If you have a history of any of these chronic health problems and are experiencing a sudden shortness of breath or other difficulty breathing, call your clinician.

Prevention

If you have a respiratory or pulmonary infection we recommend that you do breathing exercises regularly, especially if you are not as physically active as you were before your diagnosis and treatment. Breathing exercises don't mean going out and jogging around the block. Your lungs can be exercised without even getting out of bed. Even something as simple as taking a few deep breaths is good for body and soul. In addition, breathing exercises can be done at any time, anywhere, and take very little time to do (see *Nasal Congestion*, p. 168, *Cough*, p. 94, *Infection*, p. 151).

> *Regardless of what type of cancer you have, it is beneficial to do simple breathing exercises a few times every day. The simple act of yawning helps your lungs expand and open up.*

When you are having problems with your breathing, you can experience:

- Anxiety
- Dizziness
- Lightheadedness

All of these problems lead to fatigue and low energy. They can also involve hyperventilation (quick, shallow breathing). This type of breathing is exactly the opposite of what you need to do to catch your breath and feel better. When you hyperventilate, you don't get more air; instead you get more anxious and breathless. When you feel yourself begin to hyperventilate, stop what you are doing and do one of the simple exercises described here.

Remedies

BREATHING EXERCISES

If you suffer any of the problems just listed, you will especially benefit from incorporating breathing exercises into your routine. However, even people with no breathing problems benefit from these easy exercises.

Exercise 1: Simple and Short   Every few hours, pretend that you are slowly blowing up a balloon. Sit or stand up straight (put your back against the wall or lie flat on the floor if you can). Fill your lungs, and feel your chest expanding and growing larger, without raising your shoulders. Blow out the air slowly and steadily with pursed lips. See how long you can take to breathe out comfortably. The more you do this exercise, the more control you will gain over your breathing.

> *This is an excellent exercise to use in an MRI or during any procedure when you need to feel calm.*

Exercise 2: Simple and a Little Longer   Sit somewhere quiet with your back straight and supported. Close your eyes. Breathe in on a slow steady count. At first, count from one to five while you are breathing in, then work up to a longer count of up to ten. Feel your lungs expanding up to the triangles between your neck and shoulders and up above your collarbone. Hold your breath for one to two beats and then, very slowly, try to exhale on an even longer count than you breathed in on. Over time, you will gain more control over your speed and effort.

See also *Meditation,* p. 242, and *Relaxation,* p. 252, for more suggestions, including yoga.

CANCER PAIN

When dealing with pain from cancer, there are two key things to remember:

- Cancer pain is real.
- Cancer pain is not a symptom you have to endure.

Pain is a very common side effect of many cancers and cancer treatments, but you do not have to grin and bear it. Eliminating and controlling your pain is a critical component of your cancer treatment. Pain can disturb your body's healing processes as well as your ability to enjoy life. Your comfort is always important, so you need to be assertive about your comfort needs. Don't wait until pain becomes unbearable before you let your clinicians know about it. Cancer pain can literally take over your life. The sooner you begin to treat it, the easier it will be to manage pain effectively.

For pain after surgery, see *Aches and Pains,* p. 33.

For nerve pain or burning, see *Numbness and Tingling,* p. 181.

Don't Give up Trying To Get Your Pain Under Control

There is also such a thing as psychological discomfort. This isn't physical pain, but it can disturb your overall sense of well-being. If your body feels fine, but you are having trouble sleeping, eating, concentrating, or socializing, see the specific section that applies to your situation (for example, *Anger,* p. 45, *Anxiety,* p. 48, *Depression,* p. 102, *Grief,* p. 228, and *Stress,* p. 264) for suggestions on remedies. Don't hesitate to discuss your discomfort with your clinician for his or her help and input.

> *This is not a time to be stoic. Let your clinicians know about your pain, so they can help you.*

Pain is what *you* feel and describe, not what your clinicians or anyone else thinks it should be. If you tell your clinician that your pain is an eight on a scale of one to ten, it is an eight. Your clinician's job is to help you get that pain down to a three or lower.

Managing cancer pain effectively usually involves combining a number of different approaches. These can include combinations of pain medication (including opioids, analgesics, and anti-inflammatories), relaxation techniques, support groups, exercise, acupuncture, magnets, and Therapeutic Touch, as well as applications of heat and cold to painful areas.

Diagnosis and Treatment Considerations

BONE PAIN

Pain from bone metastasis can be severe, and the treatment is complicated. In addition to opioid medications and the adrenocorticoids (cortisone, hydrocortisone, dexamethasone, methyl prednisone, methyl prednisolone, prednisone, prednisilone), there are intravenous medications such as pamidronate (Aredia) for bone strengthening that can be infused to help with the pain. Ask your clinician if this might be possible for you. The NSAIDs such as ibuprofen are not helpful with bone pain and can put you at risk for gastrointestinal bleeding. See *Radiation* and *Epidurals,* below, for more approaches to bone pain.

> *Having bone ache does not necessarily mean you have metastases. If you are on filgrastim (Neupogen) or GM-CSF, see* Neutropenia, p. 178, *for more information on bone aches.*

Generally, when we discuss medication for cancer pain, we are talking about opioids and over-the-counter pain relievers.

OPIOIDS

Opioids are commonly used in controlling chronic cancer pain. For cancer pain, opioids are often mixed with the analgesic acetaminophen (Tylenol). The addition of the analgesic to the opioid often helps provide more pain relief but the acetaminophen also limits the amount of opioid you can take, so the combination may ultimately be ineffective at providing you with enough relief. Therefore, if the combined tablet dose is not providing you with enough relief, you may need a pure opioid product without the acetaminophen. Speak to your clinician about this, because analgesics such as acetaminophen are very good in helping opioids work more effectively and will probably be continued along with your opioid regimen, although in a separate formula-

> *Relief of bone pain frequently requires the expertise of a cancer pain specialist, and we recommend that you discuss with your clinicians the possibility of getting one on your treatment team.*

tion. If you have renal failure, be aware that morphine is not recommended; oxycodone, fentanyl, or hydromorphone are preferred.

Tolerance   Your body will build up a tolerance over time to the opioid dose. This means that when you stop taking the opioid, you must taper off the dose slowly, under the supervision of your clinician. It also means that the longer you take the medication, the more your dose will probably need to be increased to continue to provide you with consistent pain relief. There is no ceiling to opioid dosing with pure opioid preparations. This means that your dose is determined by how much you need to prevent and control your pain. Good management of cancer pain involves a bit of fine tuning, so don't be surprised if you need a few days to get used to certain side effects at first or if you have to change your opioid because of other side effects.

Side Effects   Any opioid will ultimately have the side effects of constipation and dry mouth. Unfortunately, there's no way to predict how you will tolerate different opioids. It is very important for your comfort that you start using a laxative as soon as you start to use an opioid for pain relief. The prevention of constipation is paramount not only to your comfort but to your health and well-being.

As for dry mouth, see *Dry Mouth*, p. 118, for suggestions on management of this problem.

Another side effect of opioids that many people find annoying is the sensation of feeling "out of it" (the clinical term for this is *sedation*). Some opioids are more sedating than others, but how you react will depend on you. Oxycodone (the opioid in Percocet) is reported to be one of the less sedating opioids, but some people report that it can still leave them feeling fuzzy. You will notice, however, that after you take it for a few days, the sedating effect of the opioid usually lessens. With the help of your clinician, you'll have to see which opioid provides you with the greatest pain relief while causing the least sedation.

> *To avoid queasiness, make sure that you take opioids with food.*

Queasiness and Nausea   Queasiness is a side effect of opioids that can be dose related, caused by taking the opioid on an empty stomach or by a particular opioid that is the wrong one for you. It is often possible to manage this side effect by modifying the dose of opioid or by switching to a different opioid. If you are experiencing nausea and recently started taking a new pain medication, the nausea is probably caused by the new medication. You can wait a day or two to see if this side effect improves, or call your clinician and see if a different medication can be used. If your nausea began when you started taking a higher dose of opioid, you may have reached your personal dosage ceiling for this particular medication. Codeine and morphine have a particular reputation for being nauseating. If you find any medication nauseating, we recommend that you let your clinicians know as soon as possible, as your pain and discomfort need to be controlled. If your opioid is changed, be sure you are changed to an equianalgesic dose of the new opioid so that your pain relief is maintained.

Allergic Reactions Allergic reactions to medications are rare. However, people do sometimes experience sensitivities that make a medication intolerable for them. If you are sensitive to a particular drug, you may have some unpleasant side effects, but when the drug is out of your system, you will be okay. An allergic reaction, on the other hand, has the potential to be life threatening. The symptoms of an allergic reaction are breaking out in hives or a rash, feeling pressure in your chest or throat, swelling of the lips and mouth, or difficulty breathing. These symptoms can happen separately, in a progression, or all

The equianalgesic dose *is the dose of the opioid that produces the same comfort effect as the dose of your previous opioid so that you do not experience discomfort. Different opioids are dosed differently, so it is important for the dose to be equally analgesic when you are switched to a different opioid. Equianalgesic doses are available on charts produced by the various manufacturers of opioids. The difference between different opioids is potency, not effectiveness. For example, when you take two tablets of oxycodone/acetaminophen (Percocet), it contains 10 milligrams of oxycodone. If you were to be switched over to morphine, the equianalgesic dose is 15 milligrams of short-acting oral morphine.*

at once. If you suddenly have any of these symptoms, stop taking the medication and call your clinician immediately and go straight to the nearest emergency room with the medication you took. If your only symptom is a rash or hives, you can take an antihistamine such as dipenhydramine (Benadryl), but call your clinician as soon as possible to discuss your reaction. If the antihistamine does not provide quick relief or if you have any of the other symptoms listed here, go to the nearest emergency room. Above all, make sure to continue drinking fluids.

Remedies

We believe wholeheartedly in the use of complementary remedies for managing symptoms. However, in the case of cancer pain, we feel strongly that the primary objective is for you to be comfortable, and usually this means that you will need conventional pain medications. For this reason, we recommend that you use the following complementary remedies in combination with conventional pain medications, not instead of them.

CONVENTIONAL MEDICATIONS

Long-Acting Opioids   Generally, cancer pain specialists recommend that for anyone who is waking up at night from pain, or anyone who requires shorter acting pain medication such as acetaminophen and oxycodone (Percocet) more than twice a day, the pain is best managed with a long-acting version of opioid for better and more consistent relief. Morphine and oxycodone have been made into sustained release preparations that are taken orally every eight to twelve hours for good overall pain control coverage. There is also a seventy-two-hour version of the opioid fentanyl (Duragesic) available in a transdermal patch that is absorbed through the skin and subcutaneous fat. This patch is primarily recommended for people who cannot swallow or digest food. Because the fentanyl patch is so long-acting, it is difficult to modify dosing quickly. At the time of this writing, a long-acting version of hydromorphone (Dilaudid) is about to be released. This will be a welcome addition to the family of long-acting opioids.

Short-Acting Opioids Short-acting opioids (immediate release opioids), often referred to as rescue doses, come in various preparations to suit different needs. Try to keep a written log to keep track of how often you need the short-acting version. This will help your clinician raise or lower your long-acting opioid dose effectively for your comfort. If you are on a fentanyl patch for long-acting medication and need a short-acting opioid for breakthrough, be sure your clinician has calculated the correct equianalgesic dose so that you are appropriately medicated. The breakthrough or rescue dose should be equal to at least one-third of your long-acting dose to be able to provide you with relief.

> *The best cancer pain control is prevention. Therefore, we recommend that you take pain medication on time. Take your short-acting (immediate release) dose when you first feel any discomfort or before you need to do an uncomfortable activity. Nip your discomfort in the bud, or prevent it before it starts.*

Breakthrough Pain Breakthrough pain is the pain experienced while you are taking long-acting opioids. This pain breaks through the long-acting opioid you are taking and makes you uncomfortable. If you are taking a long-acting version, be sure to have a short-acting opioid version on hand for treating breakthrough pain. If you can predict an activity will be painful (such as being in a car or a wound dressing change), don't be afraid to take the breakthrough medication far enough ahead of time (usually thirty to sixty minutes if you are using an oral or rectal version) so that you will feel relief before an activity to help you get through it.

If you are on a combination of long- and short-acting opioids, be sure to always have a short-acting dose or two on hand for times when the long-acting version is just not enough. Despite the official recommendations against using different opioids together (see above), your clinician may have to combine different medications to find the recipe that works best for you.

Continuous Intravenous (IV) Opioid Preparations Morphine and hydromorphone (Dilaudid) are the two opioids commonly used in a continuous IV solution. When your clinician recommends an IV opioid for pain control, this doesn't mean you are dying; IV opioids are recommended for extremely severe mouth sores, severe cancer pain that has not been well controlled with oral medication, and after most surgery. Intravenous opioids are only given in the hospital, except at the end of life, when IV opioid solutions can be hung and managed at home by a home hospice nurse or physician (see *Death and Dying*, p. 217).

Alternatives to Opioids in Pill Form   Most short-acting opioids come in a liquid version of different concentrations. If taking anything orally is a problem, it is certainly possible to try a sublingual (under the tongue), chewable, rectal, or transdermal (through the skin) version of an opioid. A rectal dose of opioid is considered equal to the oral dose of the same opioid. The subcutaneous (under the skin) dose is equal to the intravenous dose. Discuss the possibility of using alternate routes of administration with your clinician. There are pharmacists available who specialize in making individualized preparations of medications for those who cannot tolerate the commercially available versions of medication; they are called compounding pharmacists. They are often used in pediatric and hospice environments because they are ingenious in figuring out how to administer a medication. If you have problems with oral medications, try to find a compounding pharmacist. It is possible to have these types of medications shipped to you. The International Academy of Compounding Pharmacists, at (800) 927-4227, or www.compass-net.com/iacp, can provide you with a list of compounding pharmacies in the United States.

ACUPUNCTURE

Skilled acupuncturists can painlessly insert thin needles into certain points along invisible channels that are called meridians. The needles are usually kept in place for less than one-half hour. Acupuncture is simple, and research has shown it to be effective for pain relief. Acupuncture has few side effects, and the cost is low. Names of qualified acupuncturists can be obtained from the American Association of Acupuncture and Oriental Medicine, located in Pennsylvania at (610) 266-1433, or through the National Commission for the Certification of Acupuncturists in Washington, D.C., at (202) 232-1404. Many private health insurance plans and HMO plans cover acupuncture services. Contact your insurance benefits office first, however, to make sure this is covered.

We recommend that you only consult an acupuncturist who is properly licensed. Be sure to let your acupuncturist know about your cancer, and make sure the acupuncturist doesn't place needles in a tumor site. Do not have acupuncture performed if you are neutropenic, have a low white blood cell count or a low platelet count, or have just started on anticoagulation therapy. Make sure that the needles used are new and are used only once. We do not know the safety of acupuncture while on radiation treatment or two days before and after chemotherapy treatment. You may choose to avoid it at these times.

HERBAL REMEDIES

Ginger Compress   A warm compress is a traditional remedy for pain. A ginger compress combines the healing properties of wet heat and herbal medicine. To make a ginger compress, put slices of fresh ginger into a large pot of water. Heat the water for fifteen minutes without letting the mixture come to a boil. After removing the pieces of ginger, soak a cloth in the warm liquid. Wring out the cloth carefully. You may want to wear gloves to protect your hands as you do this. If the cloth is too hot, wrap it in a towel. Place the warm cloth on the site of the pain, removing it when the compress cools.

EPIDURAL PAIN RELIEF

Sometimes bone pain is too severe to be treated only with oral medication or radiation. In this situation, epidural catheters can be used to deliver pain relief directly to the spine.

MAGNETS

Although researchers do not know exactly how magnets work, in a recent study at Baylor Medical School in Houston, magnets were shown to be effective in reducing foot pain in diabetics. A study of magnets for fibromyalgia is under way at the University of Virginia. Magnets come in different shapes and sizes, including magnets to insert in your shoes, seat cushions, and mattress pads. While more research on the effectiveness of magnets in relieving pain needs to be done, the current recommendations are to use magnets with strengths of 200–1,000 gauss (slightly stronger than your basic refrigerator magnet). Typically, people do not feel any sensation from the magnets. It is advised that people with pacemakers, low platelets, or bleeding disorders should not use magnets.

MEDITATION AND RELAXATION TECHNIQUES

Meditation and relaxation techniques can be very helpful in managing cancer pain. These techniques can help you deal with the anticipation and anxiety surrounding pain as well as the pain itself. Meditation and relaxation techniques have been studied for their positive effect on pain. These techniques not only redirect your focus from your pain but also can provide you with a sense of well-being and comfort. See *Meditation,* p. 242, *Relaxation,* p. 252, and *Anxiety,* p. 48.

RADIATION FOR BONE METASTASIS

Bone metastases that are painful can also sometimes be treated with two to three weeks of radiation or even injected radioactive treatments administered in the nuclear medicine suite. The goal of these treatments is to stop the pain, control the spread of cancer in the affected area, and stabilize the bone to prevent further problems. The full comfort effect of the radiation treatments can be delayed for a week or so, so you may not feel relief immediately.

> *While a recent study published in the* Journal of the American Medical Association (JAMA) *claims that Therapeutic Touch doesn't work, other studies have shown positive effects from Therapeutic Touch, and many people have reported to have benefited from this technique over*

THERAPEUTIC TOUCH (TT)

Therapeutic Touch is a process in which the practitioner (often a nurse) uses his or her hands as a focus to redirect energy for healing. Contrary to what the name might imply, there is generally no physical touch involved. Therapeutic Touch treatments can increase a sense of well-being and decrease pain in persons with cancer. A typical Therapeutic Touch session lasts somewhere between ten and thirty minutes, during which the recipient sits or lies down fully clothed. The vast majority of patients who participate in a Therapeutic Touch session report feeling deeply relaxed during the treatment.

For more suggestions on other alternative approaches to cancer pain management, see *Aches and Pains,* p. 33.

Acetaminophen with Codeine   For cancer pain relief, acetaminophen with codeine (Tylenol 3) is considered a very poor choice. There is a high incidence of nausea and severe constipation as side effects. Unlike other opioids, codeine has a dose ceiling of 120 milligrams, beyond which it is toxic. Codeine also needs to be converted by a fully functioning liver into morphine, otherwise it is ineffective. Fifteen to twenty-five percent of Caucasians are genetically unable to metabolize codeine. For these reasons, it is agreed among most cancer clinicians that codeine is an inappropriate opioid for cancer pain.

Intramuscular Injections   Intramuscular injections of opioid are no more effective than subcutaneous, intravenous, or oral preparations, although they are considerably more painful to receive. It is considered inappropriate to treat cancer pain in a painful manner, unless there are absolutely no immediate alternatives to provide you with pain relief.

Meperidine Hydrochloride (Demerol)   Meperidine has no place in cancer pain management. Both the World Health Organization and the United States Department of Health and Human Services Agency have issued cancer pain guidelines to support this. Meperidine is not only short-acting but is only effective for a maximum of seventy-two hours. Meperidine also takes a long time to be cleared from your body and has many serious adverse effects, including seizure. It is also not recommended for the elderly because of its high incidence of neurotoxicity.

Propoxyphene (Darvon, Darvon-N, Darvocet-N)   Propoxyphene is no more effective for pain relief than two tablets of acetaminophen yet has all the side effects of other opioids. This is an inappropriate pain medication for anyone with chronic pain or cancer pain and is especially not recommended for treating any type of pain in the elderly.

COLDS

A cold is an upper respiratory viral infection. The symptoms we complain about when we have a cold, such as a cough, runny nose, and congestion, are the immune system's responses to the viral invasion, not due to the infection itself. Ironically, if you treat a cold too aggressively, you may end up prolonging it by not allowing your immune system to do its job and rid your body of the virus.

Myths about Colds

· Going outside on a cold day with wet hair does not cause colds.
· Colds are not caused by chills, bad weather, or sitting on a cold stone.

You must come in contact with the actual cold virus to get a cold. These behaviors do affect your immune system, however, by making you more vulnerable to cold viruses and less able to protect yourself.

Diagnosis and Treatment Considerations

ANTIBIOTICS

If you get a cold while you are on cancer treatment, it is not unusual for a clinician to put you on an oral antibiotic as a preventative measure to stop a secondary bacterial infection while your immune system is busy during treatment (see *Infection,* p. 151, and *Immunity,* p. 233).

FEVER

While you are on cancer treatment, fever is often a reliable guide as to whether or not you have a cold. Sometimes a person with a compromised immune system doesn't work up any symptoms except a fever as a sign of infection. See *Fever,* p. 126.

Diagnosis and Treatment Considerations

Anyone with a chronic disease needs to avoid infections. Call your clinician if you have a cold or flu and you are having a difficult time:

· Coughing
· Drinking clear fluids
· Increasing your fluids
· Sitting up
· Walking

or:

- If you are on supplemental oxygen
- If you have a temperature higher than what your clinician has told you is acceptable for you

In these instances, your clinician will probably want you to come into the office for an exam. What is just a simple cold for someone else could be very serious for you.

Prevention

While you are on any kind of cancer treatment, it is a good idea to tell anyone with a cold who wants to visit you to postpone the visit until they are feeling well. Of course, you can meet outside where there is lots of air to dilute the germs. If it's cold season, always ask people to wash their hands thoroughly before they touch you.

Hand-washing is very important because you do not want to infect or re-infect yourself by introducing the virus to your eyes, nose, or mouth.

WASH YOUR HANDS (AND OTHER TIPS)

The absolutely best prevention of a cold is to wash your hands well with a mild soap. Wash your hands before you eat anything, after you use the bathroom, after handling a newspaper, and especially after you blow your nose.

Make sure not to pick your lips or nose or chew your fingernails, especially when you have a cold. And try not to rub your eyes or touch your mouth unless you have washed your hands first. Touching your eyes with dirty hands can be a very effective way to infect yourself.

Do not kiss children under age ten on the mouth or lips or share food with them. Children have immature immune systems and therefore are excellent sources of all kinds of bacteria and

If you move between different climates throughout the day (from a hot day outside to air-conditioning, or vice versa) be sure to wear layers and a hat if necessary. This makes it easier to maintain a consistent and comfortable body temperature, making it easier on your metabolic system.

viruses. Cheek-kissing and hugs are fine, as long as the child washes his or her hands before touching you.

Be sure to get your flu vaccine every fall unless you are told to avoid it by your clinician. Be sure to ask your clinician about the pneumococcal vaccine, which is to prevent pneumonia infections for those with compromised immune systems. This vaccine is usually given every five to ten years. This vaccine is not recommended for someone undergoing treatment for Hodgkin's disease (see *Immunity*, p. 233).

Remedies

WHAT TO DO IF YOU HAVE A COLD

Increase the amount of fluids you are drinking. Don't be afraid to be on a diet of mostly fluids (just make sure you include enough calories in those fluids).

- Eat lots of warm soups and drink lots of clear liquids.
- Try drinking warm water flavored with lemon, adding honey only if you are not neutropenic. Overall, it may be best to forgo honey until after you are all done with treatment (see *Immunity*, p. 233, and *Neutropenia*, p. 178).
- Gargle frequently with saline solution to keep your mouth clean and fresh.
- Dress in layers appropriate for the weather to avoid being chilled or overheated. Layers are what is generally recommended for better and consistent body temperature control.

Remember that colds usually go away on their own accord no matter what you do to get rid of them. The most important things you can do when you are infected with a cold are to drink more fluids, take it easy, and keep your body at a steady, consistent temperature. It's important to take care of yourself when you have a cold because while you have an infection, your immune system works harder. Whenever your immune system is compromised, either by illness, disease, stress, or as a side effect of treatment, you are at a greater risk of more serious respiratory infections, as well as other infections. If your cold is getting worse instead of better after a few days, call your clinician.

AROMATHERAPY

Eucalyptus Oil   Eucalyptus oil can help relieve congestion. Put five drops into a steaming pot of water, drape a towel over your head, and carefully inhale the steam. Steam inhalation is not recommended if you are currently on radiation to the head or neck, as the wet heat can irritate your skin.

HERBAL REMEDIES

Thyme or Sage Tea   Tea made with the herbs sage or thyme can help relieve congestion and soothe the throat. You can use fresh or dried herbs.

SALINE NASAL IRRIGATION

A yoga technique that works well for cold prevention is to rinse your nostrils daily with a simple saline spray. This is called nasal irrigation. You can buy saline solution at the drugstore or make your own.

Making your own nasal saline solution is inexpensive, simple, and easy. Add half a teaspoon of table salt (or sea salt) to a quart of cold water. Heat on the stove to melt the salt; cool in a jar. You can keep this solution in the bathroom in a nasal spray bottle and use as needed.

To use your saline solution, hang your head back over the edge of a bed or a chair back, or you can also "sniff" the saline solution from the palm of your hand while pressing one nostril closed. Put ten to twelve saline drops in each nostril. When you finish, blow your nose very gently to catch any fluid or mucus. You can also use a nasal spray bottle or a bulb nasal syringe for coating the nasal passages with saline solution. Use this technique daily during cold and flu season to prevent infection.

VITAMINS AND MINERALS

Vitamin C   The best dietary sources of vitamin C are fresh citrus fruits and juices. You can also take supplemental vitamin C for colds, but we do not ever recommend megadosing. See *Immunity*, p. 233, and *Nutrition*, p. 244, for a discussion regarding taking antioxidant vitamins during chemotherapy and radiation treatment. If you are on treatment for head, neck, or esophageal cancers, or if you have mouth sores, avoid drinking fruit juice and eating citrus fruit. The citric acid will be painful and irritating to your mouth and throat.

Zinc Lozenges   Zinc lozenges are reported to help your immune system be less vulnerable to viral infections. Zinc lozenges also are used to soothe a sore throat. Some clinical studies have shown that using zinc lozenges can reduce the length and severity of colds, while other studies show no effect. As for taking zinc while on radiation, it is probably safe to ingest it while under treatment, even though it is a metal. However, if you are concerned, allow at least four hours to elapse before your radiation treatment or take the lozenge after you are done with treatment for the day. Zinc is not recommended if you are also on an adrenocorticoid (cortisone, hydrocortisone, dexamethasone, methyl prednisone, methyl prednisolone, prednisone, or prednisilone).

GARGLING

Try gargling with warm water, adding a couple of drops of tea tree oil. Always dilute tea tree oil for use in the mouth. Tea tree oil is not recommended if you have mouth sores (mucositis) or during radiation to the neck or mouth.

USE WITH CARE

Cold Remedies   Use cold remedies carefully and knowledgeably. Some symptoms may actually get worse if you try to control them instead of letting them work themselves out. If you have a symptom that is making you miserable, we recommend using only the specific remedy for that symptom. See *Cough,* p. 94, *Fever,* p. 126, or *Nasal Congestion,* p. 168. Be very careful about using over-the-counter cold and flu remedies, especially those that claim to treat multiple symptoms. If you are having trouble sleeping because of congestion, coughing, or sneezing, it is probably okay to use one of these products, but try to treat only the symptom that is bothering you. Decongestants and antihistamines work on colds and allergies by drying you out. These products don't just dry out your nose, they dry out your entire body. We recommend that you drink extra fluids if you are using any of these products. As we discussed earlier, the symptoms of a cold are your body's mechanism for trying to get rid of the virus (see *Nasal Congestion,* p. 168).

WE DO NOT RECOMMEND

Antibacterial Soaps   There are many new antibacterial products on the market right now. However, since colds and the flu are caused by viruses, not bacteria, all these antibacterial products, from soap to paper towels, are useless against colds. They are not only useless against colds, but they can be harsh on your skin and your wallet. Keeping your hands clean and your skin intact with a mild bar soap is your best defense against infection.

> *If you are achy and feeling blah, take your temperature, call your clinician, and then see* Fever, *p. 126,* Infection, *p. 151, and* Neutropenia, *p. 178.*

Echinacea and Goldenseal   These herbs are not recommended while on treatment, as either one may interfere with the effectiveness of your treatment. Goldenseal should not be combined with other anticoagulants. Echinacea should not be combined with adrenocorticoids and is not recommended after bone marrow or stem cell transplant.

Ephedra   Be very cautious if you are taking a product containing ephedra or ma huang. Ephedra is a potent heart stimulant and can be quite dangerous if you are taking other stimulants or MAO inhibitors or if you have heart problems. Ephedra can be found in many "natural" cold and allergy remedies in different forms (tea, capsule, pill, or liquid). Read the ingredients of any product you use very carefully before taking it.

Nonsaline Nasal Sprays   Only use saline nasal sprays. Other kinds of nasal cold sprays may clear your nose immediately, but ultimately they prolong your cold by not allowing your body to get rid of the virus.

For more information on the complementary remedies discussed in this section, see chapter 3.

CONCENTRATION PROBLEMS

Concentration is the ability to apply oneself to the completion of a task. Determining whether your level of concentration has been affected by your cancer or your treatment is very subjective and can only be evaluated by you. Confusion can be a related, but different, problem (see *Confusion,* p. 87). If you are concerned about your memory, see *Medication Safety and Your Memory,* p. 239.

Improving Concentration

The ability to concentrate can often be affected by other problems, including breathing problems, fatigue, nutrition problems, pain, and stress.

> *Concentration problems sometimes exist because you're having problems living with the idea of what is happening to you. See* Anger, *p. 45, and* Depression, *p. 102.*

See the individual sections on each of these symptoms for specific suggestions on their management. Relieving these symptoms can improve your ability to concentrate. Learning to use relaxation, meditation, or exercise can also help concentration (see *Exercise,* p. 223, *Meditation,* p. 242, *Relaxation,* p. 252, and *Stress,* p. 264).

Diagnosis and Treatment Considerations

Concentration is rarely a problem with an organic cause, but there are a few situations where it can be.

BRAIN TUMOR AND BRAIN METASTASIS

Depending on where the brain lesions are located, different brain functions and emotions can be affected. The treatments for brain tumors and metastases usually include radiation, chemotherapy, surgery, or a combination of these treatments. We recommend that before you start treatment, you discuss these issues in depth with your clinician so that you are comfortable about what to expect.

BONE MARROW AND STEM CELL TRANSPLANTS

There is some evidence that bone marrow and stem cell transplants can affect concentration for a year or more after you have completed the procedure. It is not entirely understood why this happens.

Remedies

AROMATHERAPY

Cardamom, Ginger, or Black Pepper Oil   To improve concentration, in her book *The Complete Book of Essential Oils and Aromatherapy,* Valerie Worwood recommends using the essential oils of ginger, cardamom, and black pepper. Use a few drops of each essential oil in equal proportions, either in a diffuser or a plant sprayer. If you use a plant sprayer, remember to dilute the essential oils in a cup of water first.

For more information on the complementary remedies discussed in this section, see chapter 3.

CONFUSION

Experiencing new, sudden, or continuing confusion is usually a sign that something is wrong. Confusion can be a sign of infection, dehydration, malnutrition, blood circulation problems, stroke, a reaction to medication, an indication of elevated levels of calcium or other electrolytes, or progression of your disease. In some cases, confusion can be caused by cancer and cancer treatment, while in other cases it is totally unrelated to cancer.

Diagnosis and Treatment Considerations

If you are older than fifty, you could be experiencing what clinicians refer to as early signs of senile dementia or Alzheimer's disease. If you have a history of extensive alcohol use, the confusion could be related to liver or kidney function. Certain chemotherapies can also interfere with liver and kidney function.

EVALUATING YOUR CONFUSION

Is this confusion a new and sudden problem? Or is it a confusion that has steadily gotten worse? If it is sudden and new, you may need to call your clinician immediately, as this can be the first sign of infection, dehydration, medication reaction, or stroke. All of these possible causes need to be taken care of as soon as possible.

Any new confusion that appears out of the blue is a reason to call your clinician. Let your clinician try to figure out what is causing the confusion. Sudden confusion can frequently be reversible if the cause can be determined and it is treated quickly.

CONSTIPATION

Constipation is something we all suffer from at one time or another, especially when we don't feel well or are taking medication. And while there are many things that are out of your control in life, constipation is something you can learn to evaluate and manage well.

Factors That Can Lead to Constipation

- Recent surgery
- Pain medications
- Chemotherapy drugs
- Antacids and GI medications
- Antihistamines and decongestants
- Antinausea medications
- Supplemental iron
- Fatigue
- A diet heavy in binding foods (bananas, rice, applesauce, dry toast, cheese)
- Diuretics
- Not enough fluid
- Not enough fiber
- Not enough physical movement
- Changes in activity level
- Changes in diet; poor diet
- Travel
- Restricted fluid prescription
- Hypercalcemia

Diagnosis and Treatment Considerations

Anal, rectal, and colon cancer patients should not use enemas or suppositories without discussing it first with their clinician.

COLON CANCER

Use remedies carefully if you have colon cancer. The most common chemotherapy regimen for colon cancer is 5-fluorouracil/leukovorin, which often causes diarrhea followed by constipation in a vicious cycle. It may be possible to modify your chemotherapy regimen, without losing its effectiveness, to help minimize this unpleasant side effect.

GASTRIC CANCER

This is a complicated type of cancer where constipation remedies are best discussed first with your doctor.

CHEMOTHERAPY

Thalidomide, Vincristine (Oncovin), Vinblastine (Velban), or Vindesine (Eldisine) If you have new constipation, new abdominal pain, and/or vomiting after eating that lasts longer than two days after administration of any of these chemotherapy medications, call your clinician immediately. Vincristine is the most likely of these to cause this problem.

Prevention

FIBER AND FLUIDS

Fiber and fluids are essential in preventing and treating constipation. Drinking large quantities of fluids every day is critical. While it can be difficult to drink enough fluid, try to drink between two and three liters of fluid per day. Consuming large quantities of fluids can be difficult when you don't feel well, or you may get full quickly. Try to do the best you can. Fluids include soup, milk shakes, and liquid nutritional supplements. If plain water is hard for you to drink, add a little juice. If you need to take antihistamines, diuretics, or medications that dry you out, you may need to drink even more fluids than you think. Many people mistakenly limit their fluid intake while on diuretics. If you are on diuretics, keep drinking fluids; otherwise you will be at risk for dehydration.

Liquids to Avoid   Coffee, black and green tea, alcohol, and caffeinated soft drinks are all mild diuretics and dry you out. Don't increase amounts of these drinks thinking that you are increasing your fluids, because they will only encourage fluid loss.

Sources of Fiber   The main sources of fiber are fresh fruits (especially the skins), certain grains (oatmeal, bran, whole cereal grains), and vegetables. If you cannot include these items in your diet, it may be necessary to take fiber as a supplement or use a laxative to preserve regularity.

Avoid Binding Foods   Binding foods are bananas, rice, applesauce, and dry toast, otherwise known as the BRAT diet, a common remedy for diarrhea. Are you eating a lot of any one or all of these foods? This may be contributing to your constipation. Cheese, cooked vegetables, peeled fruits, and stewed fruits also frequently have binding effects.

Remedies

ADD THE FOLLOWING TO YOUR DIET

- Bran in any form (forget the bran muffin; have a bowl of bran cereal)
- Yogurt with live acidophilus bacteria (most yogurts now have this, but read the label to be sure)
- Apples with skin, prunes, fresh fruit, old-fashioned cooked oatmeal (for pectin)
- Fresh or steamed vegetables (for bulk)
- Olive oil; one to two tablespoons after breakfast
- The juice of half a lemon in a cup of warm water, first thing every day

If changing your diet has no effect, we recommend that you try a combination of over-the-counter products.

Senna and Stool Softener   For those on opioids for pain relief, Senna is a laxative that stimulates the bowel. It is very well tolerated by most people. We don't recommend a combined senna/stool softener in a one-tablet version (Senakot-S, for example) unless you have problems with pills, as it will limit the amount of senna you can take. Because senna stimulates the bowel, the side effects (abdominal cramping, excessive gas, and/or diarrhea) are easy to recognize. By the way, senna is the herb cassia actufiolia and is totally natural. You may find that sometimes the senna works great and sometimes it works too well. Listen to your body. It's okay to fine-tune your dose. You can take up to a maximum of four tablets of senna four times a day. However, if you are experiencing side effects with a low dose of senna, please don't take any more. You may be better off with a different laxative. Some people find they have good control of their bowels when they skip a dose of senna. Try different combinations as long as you do not increase the amount of senna too quickly (that is, don't increase the total dose by more than two tablets daily).

Stool softener consists of docusate sodium (Colace is the most well-known brand) and is available over the counter. The capsule preparation is easiest to swallow, is not filling, and will not interfere with your absorption of nutrients. This stool softener is also available in liquid form, but we recommend it in liquid form only if you have trouble swallowing capsules. Do not exceed the label dosage of three capsules per day. Do not combine stool softener with mineral oil.

You may hear and read that senna is not good to take forever, but as it is readily available, reliable, and inexpensive, we recommend it. Your bowels will become dependent on this laxative over time, but only after a long period. If this disturbs you, try cascara sagrada (see below). Cascara is very effective and is gentler than senna, but it's also much more expensive.

You can add stool softener by itself to your daily routine if your bowel problem is only with hard stools (see *Hemorrhoids*, p. 000), but if you are taking opioids, stool softener alone will be ineffective in preventing or treating constipation.

WHEN SENNA AND STOOL SOFTENER AREN'T FOR YOU OR YOU ARE NOT ON OPIOID PAIN RELIEF

Magnesium Laxative (milk of magnesia, magnesium citrate, or magnesium sulfate)   Increasing magnesium can cause diarrhea, so for the person with constipation this may be just what is needed. We recommend these products for the occasional "get going" dose, not for maintenance, as you need to be careful about taking too much magnesium. It is not recommended that you use magnesium-based products if you are on blood pressure, cardiac, or renal medications or if you have kidney failure. Magnesium-based laxatives are also not recommended for long-term use.

Cascara Sagrada   This plant supplement can be expensive, but it is very safe to use. The dosage is one gram, which is approximately half a teaspoon of liquid extract or powder. Don't use if pregnant or nursing.

Buckthorn   Buckthorn is similar to cascara sagrada in dosage and effectiveness.

Bisacodyl (Ducolax, Fleet Lax, Dulcagen)   Bisacodyl usually works in six to ten hours. This medication can cause abdominal cramping and gas. The recommended dose is one 10- or 15-milligram tablet by mouth one to two times per day. This medication also comes in a 10-milligram rectal suppository that can work very quickly. Do not take these tablets with milk or antacids. Bisacodyl can be added to the senna/stool softener combination if it is not effective enough.

Lactulose   This syrup can be difficult to take because of its taste and consistency, but sometimes you need this strong a medicine to control constipation. Mixing the dose into fruit juice can improve the taste a little. Lactulose usually takes a few doses to be effective, but when it kicks in, the effect is often fairly explosive. Know where the bathrooms are. You can also expect some gas. Lactulose can be added every other day or every day if the senna/stool softener and bisacodyl combination is not enough. This is not recommended for diabetics.

Use with Care

We include the following remedies because people want to know about these products. The following herbal remedies work well because of how effective the bowel stimulation is, but they can cause uncomfortable abdominal cramping and are therefore not recommended for most cancer patients. These medications are not recommended for those on blood pressure or cardiac medications.

ALOE JUICE

Buy this in the liquid form (prepared professionally), which is available in many health food stores. Remember, aloe juice is different from the gel that you get directly from the plant. Do not eat a leaf from your houseplant. Aloe juice is made from the dried juice of the leaves. The gel is used externally, while aloe juice can be taken internally. Take one tablespoon of aloe juice up to three times a day.

RHUBARB ROOT

Also known as Chinese rhubarb and turkey rhubarb, this is not the same rhubarb used in pie; it is the root of the plant. Rhubarb root comes in powdered and tablet forms. In powdered form, take one teaspoon in a half cup of warm water every day. The German Commission E endorses the use of rhubarb for constipation. In smaller doses, it is also used to treat diarrhea. We do not recommend using rhubarb root for a prolonged period of time (more than three days). It is also not recommended for use by pregnant or nursing women.

We Don't Recommend

ENEMAS

Enemas need to be used with caution, especially after bowel surgery or if your blood or platelet counts are low. Only use enemas if this is really your preferred method of relieving your constipation or if you can't take things by mouth. Enemas are not recommended for those currently on pelvic radiation or anal radiation.

MINERAL OIL (FLEET MINERAL OIL, HALEY'S M-O)

Mineral oil is an excellent lubricant for the bowel when used as an enema, but taken orally, it can block the absorption of nutrients you need. Therefore, only take it on an empty stomach, at least one-half hour before eating. Mineral oil is not used at bedtime, as bowel activity slows during sleep. Do not combine mineral oil with ducosate sodium (Colace).

PSYLLIUM

We do not recommend psyllium seed preparations (Citrucel, Metamucil) for most cancer patients with constipation. Psyllium seed laxatives require additional fluid immediately with the dose, and it can be very difficult to maintain enough fluid every day. Sometimes psyllium is used to help people with diarrhea problems, since it can bulk the stool up so well.

For more information on the complementary remedies discussed in this section, see chapter 3.

COUGH

It may be helpful to understand that a cough is your body's mechanism to keep your airway clear. It is completely normal to cough once in a while. It is a common way to clear your throat in the morning or react to an irritant such as dry air.

> *Coughs can be infectious or noninfectious. Infectious coughs are a problem not only for you but for everyone around you. We recommended that you always cover your mouth when you cough and wash your hands with soap afterward.*

Causes

RESPIRATORY INFECTIONS

Unfortunately, there are also a couple of nasty respiratory infections that can cause coughs and are quite serious. These include tuberculosis (TB) and pneumonia, which are very serious public health problems. You are unlikely to have tuberculosis unless you have been directly exposed to it in concentrated amounts over a period of time. If you find out you have been exposed to TB, be sure to tell your clinician, and a simple skin test can be done to determine if you have the disease. Pneumonia, on the other hand, is fairly common but can still be stressful and debilitating, especially when your body is already busy dealing with everything else. The hallmark signs of bacterial or viral pneumonia are a bad, deep cough that hurts in your chest, a loss of appetite, and profound fatigue, with or without a fever. If this is how you feel, call your clinician.

> *Warning*
> *If you have a cough that is:*
> *· Very wet and frothy sounding*
> *· Occurs and increases with activity (as opposed to when you are resting)*
> *· Accompanied by shortness of breath and/or heart palpitations*
> *Call your clinician immediately.*

If you have a respiratory infection, your immune system is using the cough to try to get rid of the infectious offender. This means that controlling or suppressing your cough may not be the best approach because it could prolong your infection. There are certainly levels of tolerance, however, and we encourage you to ask your clinician for help if you believe your cough is the result of an infection.

NONINFECTIOUS

Coughing can be a side effect of a few medications. If your cough began at the same time you started taking a new medication, call the clinician who prescribed or recommended this medication to you.

Other causes of cough that are completely unrelated to cancer can include chronic lung diseases (chronic obstructive pulmonary disease, emphysema, or asthma). If you have this type of cough, you may need a pulmonary disease specialist who is an expert in the proper medications for the particular problem that is triggering your cough (see *Breathing Problems,* p. 67).

DRY MOUTH

Dry mouth can make you cough because of irritation to your mucous membranes. Dry mouth can also be accompanied by thickened saliva that collects at the back of your throat like a lump, making it difficult to swallow (see *Dry Mouth,* p. 118).

If you are not drinking enough fluids, the mucous membranes of your mouth and throat can become irritated and dried out (see *Dehydration,* p. 99).

Diagnosis and Treatment Considerations

CHEMOTHERAPY

Cladribine (Leustatin)—cough is a possible side effect.

RADIATION

Radiation to the mouth, neck, or upper center of the chest (where the esophagus is) can irritate them. The irritation is frequently expressed as a cough.

Prevention

The best way to get sick, besides not washing your hands before eating, is to hang out in a small, crowded, enclosed space with little fresh air (like a subway car, an airplane, or a room with the windows closed) with a hacking, sneezing companion (see *Colds,* p. 79). This does not mean that you should never take a subway or airplane; it just means that you need fresh air to keep the bacteria and viruses diluted. People in Japan wear cotton gloves and face masks when they have a cold and go out in public. This is not a bad idea, as it keeps people from spreading their germs via their hands. Wash your hands as soon as you can after having been in an enclosed space, and try to limit the amount of time you spend in enclosed areas.

DRY AIR

Dry air can cause coughing because it irritates your mucous membranes and lungs by drying them out. It is very important to stay hydrated to keep your secretions thin and easier to cough up. If you have forced air heat in the winter or live in an arid climate like the desert, you may need to use a cool air humidifier and drink even more than two to three liters of fluids every day.

SMOKE

Any smoke is an irritant to the mucous membranes. This includes smoke from woodstoves, fireplaces, and incense, as well as tobacco products. Try to avoid exposure to these as much as possible. If you cannot quit smoking or avoid smoke entirely, at least limit the amount of time you spend in smoky rooms.

Remedies

TREATING COUGHS

If you believe your cough is related to a new medication, you must find out from your clinician what to do. If the cough is from dry mouth, dry air, or dust, you will need to change your environment by adding moisture.

There seem to be a multitude of cough products available on the market. Be sure to read labels carefully and purchase the one that deals with your symptoms specifically. More is not better in this situation. You don't want a product that covers every possible cold symptom when you don't need it.

For a noninfectious cough that just won't go away, or one that keeps you from sleeping, a cough suppressant medicine containing an opioid, or an opioid by itself, may be the best option for you. The opioid helps to suppress the cough and will provide you with some relief. Consult your clinician for the right prescription for you.

AROMATHERAPY

Eucalyptus or Tea Tree Oil Try putting a few drops of eucalyptus or tea tree oil in your humidifier to clear your congestion and refresh the air.

CONVENTIONAL COUGH MEDICATIONS

Follow these guidelines to determine which ingredient would be the most useful to use to treat your cough, but always discuss your medications with your clinician before taking them. In addition, be aware that alcohol, which is frequently included in cough products for its sedating effect, can be drying and further irritating to your mucous membranes. We recommend that you try to find products that do not have alcohol. Pediatric versions often are alcohol free, but you must check the ingredients label.

Dextromethorphan Hydrobromide An antitussive, this works on your central nervous system to suppress the cough reflex.

Diphenhydramine A cough suppressant and antihistamine, this dries up secretions and therefore suppresses the cough by stopping the irritation. Antihistamines are generally sedating, and you should heed the warnings regarding the dangers about using them combined with operating heavy machinery (i.e., driving a car).

> *Antitussives suppress coughing and help you sleep or rest.*

Guafenesin An expectorant, this helps to thin mucus secretions.

OPIOIDS

Opioids can work well for cough management by depressing the respiratory system just enough so that you don't breathe quite as deeply, therefore suppressing the cough. Opioids are also effective in helping to dry up your secretions. If your cough is due to primary lung cancer or lung metastases, an opioid can lessen your coughing and keep you more comfortable.

Terpin Hydrate An expectorant and antitussive, this helps to thin mucus secretions and works on your central nervous system to suppress the cough reflex.

> *If you are not able to rest or sleep from your cough, try a combination of an expectorant, which helps you to cough secretions out, and an antitussive cough suppressant.*

HERBAL ANTITUSSIVE REMEDIES

Marshmallow Root, Mullein Flowers, English Plantain   Try making a soothing tea from any of these herbs. Have one cup in the evening. If you are taking digoxin (Lanoxin), plantain is not recommended, as there may be an interaction.

Slippery Elm Lozenges   Slippery elm is derived from the inner bark of the slippery elm tree. Lozenges are the most effective form of this herb and are found in health food stores. Sucking on one of these lozenges is soothing to your sore throat and upper intestinal tract. According to the FDA, slippery elm is a safe and effective soothing agent (demulcent) for treating sore throats.

MASSAGE

You can use a few drops of eucalyptus oil or thyme oil (diluted in one tablespoon of unscented oil) for a soothing chest massage. We do not recommend massage of the skin in a current radiation treatment field.

NUTRITION

Pineapple   Pineapple contains the therapeutic compound bromelain, which helps to thin out mucus, making it less cough-provoking. You can drink the juice or eat the fruit. Pineapple juice is delicious and soothing when drunk warm as a toddy.

OTHER APPROACHES TO MANAGE COUGH

We suggest using a humidifier to soothe your irritated bronchial tubes. Depending on the time of year and your preference, you can use either a warm or cool air humidifier. Be sure to clean out the reservoir frequently to prevent the buildup of mineral deposits and mold.

WE DON'T RECOMMEND

Uncooked Honey   If you are neutropenic (see *Neutropenia*, p. 178) or have recently had chemotherapy, we don't recommend using honey. Honey can have the botulinium toxin in it, which can be life threatening for those with compromised immune systems.

For more information on the complementary remedies discussed in this section, see chapter 3.

DEHYDRATION

An easy problem to develop, dehydration is also an easy one to overlook. Since 60 percent of your body consists of water, you are completely dependent on having enough fluid for your systems to function effectively. Almost every remedy in this book recommends drinking fluids because fluids serve many important purposes in your body. They help your body to get rid of waste products that are created by chemotherapy and other medications, as well as the waste from the body's own metabolic processes. They also help maintain the appropriate temperature for your body. When you don't drink enough fluids, serious problems occur (see *Constipation*, p. 88, *Diarrhea*, p. 109, *Breathing Problems*, p. 67, *Nausea and Vomiting*, p. 170).

> *If you are exercising, you need to replace the fluids you lose through sweating, in addition to drinking your normal two to three liters of fluid a day.*

Dehydration, even so-called minor dehydration, can make your blood counts appear higher in test results than they actually are because your blood becomes more concentrated (see *Anemia*, p. 40, *Neutropenia*, p. 178, *Bleeding and Bruising*, p. 61). We know that drinking two to three liters of fluid a day is not easy, but there are strategies for making it easier to accomplish, and if you make the effort, you will probably drink more than you did before. Remember, by the time you feel thirsty, your body already needs fluid, so it is important to make constant fluid intake a part of your daily routine.

> *When you are in certain situations, you need to be especially aware of how much you are drinking. For example, if you are flying in an airplane, spending a lot of time in air-conditioning or in extreme changes of temperature, your need for fluids will increase.*

General Signs and Symptoms of Dehydration

- Dry mouth and eyes
- Dry, brittle, loose, "wrinkly" skin
- Constipation
- Fever and chills

- Shakiness
- Small amounts of dark-colored urine
- Dizziness when changing positions (from lying to sitting, or from sitting to standing)
- Shortness of breath
- Confusion

Call your clinician immediately

- If you are unable to drink or eat for twelve to twenty-four hours
- If you have fever greater than 100.5 degrees F, especially if the fever is accompanied by chills
- If you have severe nausea and/or vomiting (see also *Nausea and Vomiting*, p. 170)
- If you have new diarrhea more than three times in a row and anti-diarrhea remedies are not stopping it

Diagnosis and Treatment Considerations

CHEMOTHERAPY

Cisplatin (Platinol) and Cyclophosphamide (Cytoxan)   When you are on cisplatin and cyclophosphamide, you may need even more fluid to help flush the chemicals out of your body. Your clinician may advise you to come in for intravenous "fluid replacement." You still need to try to drink as much as you can because fluid, like most nutrients, is best absorbed and utilized by your body when taken by mouth.

Prevention and Remedies

If you are taking diuretics (water pills) for blood pressure management, be sure to let your clinician know about this medication before you start cancer treatment. It is a good idea to bring all your medications (in their original bottles with the labels) to your consultation so your clinician can review them. Diuretics are for circulation problems, not because you drink too much fluid.

Fluids

HOW MUCH IS ENOUGH?

We recommend drinking two to three liters of fluid a day. While it can be difficult to drink enough fluid, do the best you can. You may get full quickly, but if you spread your consumption of liquids throughout the day, you may find it easier to get in those two to three liters. Remember that fluid includes soup, milk shakes, and liquid nutritional supplements. If plain water is hard for you to drink, add a little juice. An excellent approach to being sure you are drinking enough is to use a "sippy cup" with a top. Make sure you know the liquid measure of your cup. You can carry it around with you and drink from it all day, filling it up as necessary until you reach the recommended two to three liters. You will drink more if you are sipping frequently. Another strategy is to use an old one-quart or one-liter soda bottle as a decanter and decant from it all day. You will be able to measure how much you really are drinking this way if you only decant your fluids from the measurable bottle. You need to drink two to three bottles' worth every day.

> *If you need to take antihistamines or other medications that have the side effect of drying you out, you may need to drink even more! Perhaps there is another medication with the desired effect that you can take instead of the one that dries you out.*

If drinking fluid is difficult, try to drink on a schedule, an eight-ounce glass every hour. Treat fluid as a medicine instead of a thirst quencher. This method is especially effective in winter or when you are less active.

We Don't Recommend

DIURETICS

Coffee, Green or Black Tea, and Caffeinated Soft Drinks   People may not realize they are dehydrated if they are drinking large amounts of coffee and green or black tea. They believe they are getting fluids, but they are actually drinking much less fluid than they think. Coffee, tea, alcohol, and caffeinated soft drinks are all diuretics. These liquids dry you out. It's okay to have your usual cappuccino or iced tea every day, but don't be fooled into thinking that these fluids are part of your fluid count.

HERBS

If you are having problems with dehydration or with getting enough fluid, we suggest that you avoid the following herbs, as they act as diuretics:

- Dandelion
- Parsley
- Uva ursi
- Nettle
- Dong quai

For more information on the complementary remedies discussed in this section, see chapter 3.

DEPRESSION

We all experience depression at one time or another in our lives. When you are depressed, you may feel sad or empty or just simply stop taking pleasure in living. Depression is a normal part of living when experienced occasionally and when you are able to recover quickly from the depressed feeling. But when this feeling lingers, it is something to pay attention to. Because wellness applies to your body and your mind, improving your mental state does more than make you feel better; it also appears to enhance the ability of your immune system to deal with your cancer and treatment.

Depression is complicated. As any good psychotherapist will tell you, depression is not just in the mind but affects the whole body. It can be difficult to differentiate the effects of fatigue, lack of appetite, poor energy levels, and sadness from the effects of being depressed. Trust your intuition. If you think you are depressed, you probably are.

Some cancer-related events—finding out you have a diagnosis of cancer,

Depression can become a vicious cycle. Being depressed can lead to isolating yourself and avoiding your ordinary activities, which can lead to feeling more depressed. The earlier you get help to try to manage these feelings, the sooner you will feel better.

trying to understand and make decisions about your treatment options, having setbacks in terms of your cancer and treatment—are depressing and are guaranteed to have a negative effect on your mood and self-image. That said, we want to reassure you that having a diagnosis of cancer does not mean you are supposed to suffer with depression. If you are feeling low, you can get help to make yourself feel better. If you are depressed, and the sadness lingers, we encourage you to seek professional help. When you are depressed, it is hard to believe there is a way out. A therapist or counselor can help you find your way back to hope.

Diagnosis and Treatment Considerations

You may not be aware of this, but there are many medications that can enhance feelings of depression or cause depression chemically. We advocate that you carefully read the information given with any drug you are taking to see if depression is a known side effect. If the drug you are taking doesn't come with information, ask for it. If you've just started taking a new medication and have begun to feel depressed, the depression may very well be a side effect of the new medication. Ask your doctor if there is another medication you could take instead. You don't have to suffer needlessly. Remember, you have options.

CHEMOTHERAPIES THAT CAN CAUSE DEPRESSION

- Vincristine (Oncovin)
- Vinblastine (Velban)
- Procarbazine (Elspar)
- Asparaginase
- Ifosfamide (Ifex)
- Interferon alpha (Roferon, Intron A)

OTHER MEDICATIONS WITH DEPRESSION AS A SIDE EFFECT

- Adrenocorticoids (cortisone, hydrocortisone, dexamethasone, methyl prednisone, methyl prednisolone, prednisone, prednisilone)
- Sleep aids and antianxiety medications (lorazepam et al.)
- Amphotericin B—an antifungal
- Propranolol—a common cardiac medication
- Methyldopa—used in Parkinson's disease

- Drinking too much coffee or green or black tea
- Alcohol consumption
- Being dehydrated
- Not getting restful sleep
- Having a poor appetite

WAS THIS A PROBLEM BEFORE DIAGNOSIS?

If you have a history of depression, it is more than likely that hearing a diagnosis of cancer will trigger a period of depression. Think about what has worked in the past to help get you through your depression. If you have gone to a therapist in the past whom you found helpful, make an appointment and tell him or her about your diagnosis so you can be seen in a timely manner. If certain people were helpful before, contact them again. There is nothing shameful about seeking help for a problem, even if it's a problem you have had before.

Remedies

If you believe one or more of your medications are making you depressed, find out if there is an alternative medication for you to take.

Try addressing some of the other factors listed earlier that may be causing your depression. Cut back on coffee and alcohol, and try some of our remedies for insomnia or poor appetite (see *Sleep Problems*, p. 192, and *Appetite Problems*, p. 57).

If you need a more individualized approach, see your doctor and get a referral to a mental health therapist and possibly a prescription for an antidepressant. There is nothing shameful in taking medication for depression. Remember, if you had a broken leg, you'd ask for help, and depression is a reasonable problem, for which there are a variety of solutions. We cannot sing the praises of a good mental health therapist loudly enough. Everyone can use someone objective to talk to about how things are going, how they feel, and what they're afraid of, and the right therapist can be that person.

AROMATHERAPY AND MASSAGE

As a culture, we are tuned in to smells, hence the popularity of perfumes and creams. Aromatherapy is often used in combination with massage, which provides you with the additional benefit of touch. If you go for a massage, be sure to tell the massage therapist your diagnosis and consider sharing any of your symptoms to see if he or she can help you. If you can't afford or don't have access to a massage therapist, ask a friend or partner to give you a massage. It is recommended that you do not have your tumor site massaged.

Bergamot, Chamomile, Geranium, Lemon, or Rose Oil For depression, some recommended aromatherapy oils are geranium, bergamot, rose, lemon, and chamomile. If you are currently on treatment, geranium is not recommended, as it may overstimulate your immune system.

BACH FLOWER REMEDIES

Mustard—for gloom and despair
Gorse—for hopelessness
Sweet chestnut—for deep despair

As with most remedies for depression, the flower essences do not work overnight.

EXERCISE

Taking a simple walk or getting out of bed can help to produce a change in your mood. Ongoing research is proving the value of daily moderate exercise for well-being and health. Try to work yourself up to taking a walk of one mile or more daily, and see if some physical movement helps you to sleep, eat, and feel better. An added benefit of exercise is that it helps your bowels stay regular.

HERBAL REMEDIES

Ginseng If the main symptom of your depression is fatigue, you may want to try ginseng, an ancient Chinese remedy. Heavily studied, ginseng has been shown to enhance the immune system and relieve fatigue. There are many types of ginseng on the market. We recommend Siberian ginseng (eleuthero) to increase energy and reduce stress. Do make sure to buy a reputable brand, which has a standardized ginseng extract containing pure ginseng with no other ingredients, and take 100 milligrams twice a day. Try taking ginseng

Ginseng has been used in healing since the first century A.D. Its unusual shape and energizing properties have led to its renown as an aphrodisiac. It also has shown promise as a complementary therapy for fatigue when given to people undergoing chemotherapy and radiation.

for two weeks, then taking a week off. Ginseng is not recommended if you have diarrhea, poor sleep, high blood pressure, or diabetes. Ginseng is also not recommended if you are taking antihypertensive medications, antipsychotic drugs, or digoxin. There is some evidence that ginseng may have estrogenic effects and that it may therefore not be safe for women with a history of breast or endometrial cancer.

Ginkgo Biloba Commonly prescribed in Europe, ginkgo is recommended for treatment of depression in people over the age of fifty, as it may help to increase blood flow and circulation to the brain. It may also stop memory loss. The commonly recommended dosage of ginkgo is 120–240 milligrams per day. Ginkgo is not recommended for those on blood thinners or anticoagulants—aspirin, warfarin (Coumadin), heparin, feverfew, or garlic.

S-adenosyl Methionine (SAM-e) This drug (pronounced "Sammy") is a synthetic form of a compound consisting of methionine and adenosine triphosphate, which occur naturally in the body. The theory is that depressed people are low in this substance. Clinical studies have found SAM-e to be as effective against depression as some prescription antidepressants, without the same side effects. However, as this is a new product and researchers are not sure of its long-term effects, we urge you to be cautious with SAM-e. Speak to your clinician if you are interested in trying it. SAM-e is not recommended if you have a bipolar disorder or any type of anxiety disorder. Another drawback to SAM-e is the cost, which is approximately one dollar a pill.

JOURNAL WRITING

To help put things in perspective for you, even five minutes a day of writing in a journal can make a difference. There are workshops on journal writing and books on journal writing, or you can just get a notebook and start to write.

MEDITATION AND BREATHING

We all take breathing for granted, but meditation and breathing exercises can be extremely helpful when you are feeling depressed. Your breath is a powerful force in your body and can make profound changes in your mood level. Try breathing slowly and deeply for a few minutes and see how you feel. And turn to the sections on *Breathing Problems*, p. 67, *Meditation*, p. 242, and *Relaxation*, p. 252, for more suggestions.

SUPPORT GROUPS

Support groups can offer understanding and advice from other people who are having a similar experience. There are many different types of support groups. You can get a list of disease-specific associations and support groups from the American Cancer Society (1-800-ACS-2345). If you feel up to it, start your own group. You can see if there is an interest by contacting local pharmacies, local hospitals and health centers, your local library or a hospice or by talking to visiting nurses. We recommend you consider including a facilitator who is not a member of the group but can help to focus discussion and maintain ground rules. For information on how to set up your own support group, a good resource is the American Self-Help Clearinghouse, which you can reach at (201) 625-7101 for advice and publications.

> *Many studies have been published that show that going to a support group can increase the quality of life of cancer survivors. Talking to others about your feelings about your treatment and your life has been consistently shown to have a positive effect on survival time.*

VITAMINS AND MINERALS

Nutrition can have a big impact on depression, so if you are having trouble eating, it is very important to be sure you have enough nutrients and calories.

B-complex Vitamins B-complex vitamins have been linked with relieving mild depression. Try adding a B50 complex as a daily supplement to your diet. If you are over sixty, get your serum B_{12} levels checked by your clinician.

Folic Acid and Folate Low folic acid levels have also been linked with depression. Try adding 400 micrograms of folic acid daily. B-complex vitamins and folic acid may be effective together to combat mild depression. Folic acid supplementation is not recommended when you are on methotrexate or leucovorin. See *Nutrition,* p. 244.

Multivitamins Sometimes all you need is a boost to your diet and a multivitamin can do it. Many multivitamins are now designed to be appropriate to age, and there are special formulas for stress and specific conditions. Read the labels and get the right one for you. Although a multivitamin is probably safe, we don't recommend taking huge doses of vitamins without the supervision of a registered nutritionist.

USE WITH CAUTION

St. John's Wort (Hypericum Perforatum) You have probably heard about this herbal medicine, which has been shown to be effective in clinical trials for those with mild to moderate depression. If you would like to try this herbal remedy, we recommend taking St. John's wort three times a day, preferably in the form of a standardized liquid extract or powder capsule containing 0.2–1.0 milligram of hypericin (the active ingredient). Don't take more than 3 milligrams of hypericin in a day. You will probably not feel results immediately, because St. John's wort, like many prescription antidepressants, can take from four to six weeks to give results. Fair-skinned people may experience extra sensitivity to the sun while taking this herb; be sure to use a sunblock when you are outside. We do not recommend combining St. John's wort with cyclosporine, antidepressant medications, especially MAO inhibitors, or with the chemotherapies etoposide (VP-16), irinotecan (Camptosar), or topotecan (Hycamptin), as it may interfere with the chemotherapy's effectiveness. It is also recommended that you stop taking St. John's wort three weeks before surgery, as it may interfere with general anesthesia.

In chemical studies of St. John's wort, compounds similar to MAO inhibitors have been found; therefore it is advised that until more is known about this herb you take the same precautions as with MAO inhibitors—that is, do not combine St. John's wort with cold, flu, or allergy medications, adrenocorticoids, opioids, alcohol, fava beans, aged cheeses, or other foods containing tyramine.

For more information on the complementary remedies discussed in this section, see chapter 3.

DIARRHEA

Diarrhea is when you are moving your bowels too frequently or your usually firmer bowel movements are consistently too soft.

Diarrhea can be a symptom of cancer treatment, or it can be totally unrelated to your cancer. Either way, it is usually unpleasant. This section is intended to help you figure out the cause of your diarrhea and let you know what you can do for relief, and under what circumstances you are advised to call your clinician. If the approach you choose isn't working within one day, we recommend that you call your clinician. Diarrhea can quickly become a serious problem.

Diarrhea can be cause for concern because it is a sign of a rapid loss of fluid. Because diarrhea usually makes you feel awful, you don't drink or eat enough and run the risk of dehydration. Some people mistakenly believe that they should limit their fluid intake in order to slow down the diarrhea, but you should do just the opposite. We strongly recommend that you do not stop drinking fluids or eating because you have diarrhea. You can actually end up in the hospital before you realize you are severely dehydrated.

Diagnosis and Treatment Considerations

If you are on treatment for one of the following cancers, you are likely to experience diarrhea:

- Gastric (stomach)
- Colon
- Rectal
- Anal
- Ovarian
- Endometrial
- Cervical
- Prostate
- Non-Hodgkin's lymphoma (involving abdomen and/or pelvis)

If your diarrhea is new and accompanied by any of the following: bleeding, fever, chills, vomiting, pain, or new abdominal swelling—call your clinician. If you have Crohn's disease, ulcerative colitis, diverticulitis, irritable bowel syndrome (IBS), or diabetes, please discuss diarrhea management with your clinician before you start treatment.

SURGERY

Stomach or Bowel Resection Surgery   The mechanics of your intestines can change depending on the type of surgery you have had and how much intestinal tissue was removed. Ask the surgeon what you can expect in the way of side effects, such as diarrhea, after your surgery, and ask for a referral to a nutritionist before your surgery so you can learn how to modify your diet to minimize any bowel problems. If you are going to have radiation or chemotherapy after bowel surgery, it is a good idea to address future dietary strategies with a nutritionist before you get started on treatment.

Pelvic Surgery   If your treatment plan includes radiation after lower abdominal or pelvic surgery, be aware that there are surgical techniques that can be used to help protect your bowel from the radiation. Discuss the possibility of using one of these techniques with your surgeon before you have the surgery.

GRAFT VERSUS HOST DISEASE (GVHD)

This disease is a problem for people who have had nonautologous bone marrow transplants. If you have had or will have a nonautologous bone marrow transplant, we strongly recommend that you discuss diarrhea management with your bone marrow transplant team.

RADIATION TO THE ABDOMEN AND/OR PELVIS

Not all people have diarrhea as a side effect of radiation to the abdomen and/or pelvis. Whether or not you will have diarrhea, and the severity, depends on the accumulated dose of the radiation as well as your individual response to it.

Acute Diarrhea from Radiation   This kind of diarrhea gets progressively worse as your total dose of radiation increases. This means the more radiation treatments, the worse the diarrhea. Diarrhea will usually occur two to three weeks into treatment and can continue for about two to three weeks after all your radiation treatments are completed. It will start to improve after this point, but it may take three months or so for your bowel movement pattern to get back to normal.

WHAT TO DO FOR RADIATION-INDUCED DIARRHEA

We recommend that you make a plan with the help of your clinician regarding when to take antidiarrheal medications and which ones to use.

Start a low-residue diet (see box below) when you start your radiation treatments to keep bowel movements moving daily, but slowly. Drink, drink, drink. And then drink some more. You may need to go into your clinician's office for intravenous fluid to prevent dehydration. It is also not unusual to need a break from treatment if the diarrhea is getting severe.

If you are getting pelvic radiation, drink water about twenty minutes before your radiation treatment and resist going to the toilet so that you get treated with a full bladder. A full bladder can help to push the bowel up and out of the treatment field and prevent inadvertent bowel irritation.

Don't be afraid to use loperamide (Immodium) or kaolin/pectin (Kaopectate) to control more frequent stools. Don't wait until your stool is completely liquid and you are going to the bathroom five times a day to recognize diarrhea. If the over-the-counter medications are not working, there are other antidiarrheal remedies available by prescription. For example, deodorized tincture of opium (DTO, Paregoric) can be just the thing for the diarrhea equivalent of the "dry heaves" (a common problem with external beam radiation for cervical cancer).

Chronic Diarrhea from Radiation   This is a late effect caused by radiation that happens at least six months after radiation treatment. If you had radiation treatment and your diarrhea cannot be explained by any of the causes listed here, call your clinician. If it has been some time since your cancer treatment, remind the clinician that you have had radiation to the abdomen or pelvis area. There are some rare, long-term problems that can occur after radiation to these areas that may need to be taken care of before they get worse.

> *A low-residue diet limits the amount of fiber in your diet. When you limit fiber, you also lower the stimulation of your lower intestinal tract. The idea is to limit but not eliminate fiber. We recommend that you seek out the expertise of a registered dietician or nutritionist for an individualized low-residue diet. On a low-reside diet, you cook all vegetables, peel the fruit you eat, and keep consumption of dairy products and whole grains to a minimum. Keep flavoring bland. Avoid corn, in any form, and legumes like peas and nuts (see* Nutrition, *p. 244).*

CHEMOTHERAPY AND ANTIHORMONE THERAPIES

The following is a list of the chemotherapies most often associated with a side effect of diarrhea, especially when in combination with radiation to the abdomen and/or pelvis.

5-fluorouracil (5FU)   People usually experience more diarrhea when they are given this chemotherapy in combination with leucovorin or levamisole.

Methotrexate   Don't ignore diarrhea if you are on this chemotherapy, even if you are only on a very small dose. Prevent more complications by addressing diarrhea immediately with your clinician.

Irinotecan (Camptosar)   Diarrhea with this chemotherapy can be sudden and severe and needs to be treated immediately. The manufacturer warns that diarrhea can occur while you are getting the medication. However, even if you don't have any diarrhea during the infusion, the manufacturer also recommends that you take an antidiarrheal such as loperamide (Immodium) or kaolin/pectin (Kaopectate) at the first sign of abdominal cramping and at bedtime the evening you get the treatment.

Dactinomycin, Doxorubicin (Adriamycin), Docetaxel (Taxotere), Vinorelbine (Navelbine)   Diarrhea is rare with these chemotherapies, but it can be severe for some people. This diarrhea may be made more of a problem because of diet changes due to mouth sores.

Carboplatin, Anastrazole (Arimidex), Bicalutamide (Casodex)   Diarrhea has been reported but is extremely uncommon as a side effect.

NON-RADIATION-INDUCED DIARRHEA MANAGEMENT REGIMEN

The goal for managing diarrhea from chemotherapy is the same as with radiation-induced diarrhea: to prevent fluid loss and dehydration. If you will be getting one of the chemotherapies or antihormone therapies listed earlier, it is a good idea to have a diarrhea management plan ready to put into action. Hopefully, you won't need it, but be prepared anyway by working one out with your clinician.

With non-radiation-induced diarrhea, there are two basic categories: early and late. Early diarrhea occurs within the first twenty-four hours of your treatment. Late diarrhea starts twenty-four hours after your treatment.

Early Diarrhea   With early diarrhea, a prescription medication such as diphenoxylate hydrochloride/atropine (Lomotil) is usually more effective than over-the-counter antidiarrheals such as loperamide (Immodium) and kaolin/pectin (Kaopectate).

We recommend that you be aggressive with your antidiarrhea plan and use it at the first sign of abdominal cramping or softer bowel movements.

Late Diarrhea   Late diarrhea is usually well managed with the over-the-counter antidiarrheals such as loperamide (Immodium) or kaolin/pectin (Kaopectate). Use the prescription antidiarrheals for backup when the over-the-counter medication isn't helping you.

As in the case of laxatives, there are a number of different antidiarrheal medications. You may need to try different approaches. Some people find that only paregoric works, so then they don't bother with the loperamide. Or you may have a personal preference. The important thing is to discuss your plan with your clinician, follow directions, and not exceed the recommended dosage. Call your clinician immediately if you are having more than seven to nine episodes of diarrhea in a day or if you are unable to drink enough fluid.

> *If you are taking narcotics for pain management, you may not need as aggressive an antidiarrheal plan; the narcotics may actually help with diarrhea prevention because of their side effect of constipation.*

OTHER CAUSES OF DIARRHEA

Bowel Infection or Food Poisoning   If you suspect that your diarrhea is from food poisoning or a bowel infection, and you are not on any of the treatments discussed earlier, we recommend that you do not take any antidiarrheals. Your body is using the diarrhea to clean out the offending toxins. It is important to let your body do this. Keep drinking and eating to replace the fluids and nutrients you are losing. If you are currently on cancer treatment and suspect bowel infection or food poisoning, however, call your clinician immediately.

Constipation   If you've had a couple of days of constipation and then have diarrhea, the cause of your diarrhea may in fact be constipation or hard stool that is blocking your rectum. This is an extremely common problem for people who are taking opioids for pain without laxatives. In this case, refer to *Constipation,* p. 88, and *Cancer Pain,* p. 69. You may need an enema or rectal suppositories to deal with this, but be sure your blood counts and platelets are okay first.

Overuse of Laxatives   This could include overuse of fiber, coffee, or tea. Discuss this possible cause of diarrhea with your clinician to modify your constipation prevention regimen. There is no rule that says you must take laxatives the same way every day. You can take more or less depending on your needs. Most likely, your clinician will recommend that you cut back on the offending agent and increase fluids (water, juice, and sports drinks without caffeine), and you should return to your normal pattern in about forty-eight hours.

Sorbitol   You may not know it, but if you are taking commercially prepared liquefied medications and elixirs because you can't swallow pills or are using a feeding tube, you may be getting too much of this additive. The recommended limit of sorbitol is 20 grams per day, which can usually be maxed out in just one dose of any one of the liquid medications. Check the nonactive ingredients list. The amount of sorbitol will not be listed, but if it is listed as an ingredient, you can try to change formulations.

Magnesium-Containing Antacids   Stop taking them. Try a different antacid preparation that doesn't have magnesium in it (see *Heartburn,* p. 135). Magnesium is commonly used as a laxative, and it may be too much for you right now.

Low-Residue or Fiber-Restricted Diet   With radiation to the abdomen/pelvis or after bowel surgery, it is recommend that you be on a low-residue diet, which provides you with a minimal amount of bulk but not too much. This can make for softer, looser stools. Be sure you are drinking enough. If your treatment is completed, ask your clinician if you still need to be on the low residue diet. See *Nutrition,* p. 244.

OTHER RECOMMENDATIONS

If you know from your past experience that you will always have a day or two of diarrhea after your chemotherapy treatment, no matter what you do, try to load up with a couple of good meals and snacks before you get the treatment. Eat high-calorie, high-protein foods so that the nutrients are available to you after your treatment when you don't feel so well.

Remember to drink your fluids. Use a bottle you know the volume of, such as a juice or soda bottle, so that you know how much you are drinking in a day. Two quarts or two liters of liquid is the minimum amount of daily fluid we recommend. Your urine should be as clear as possible. Although we don't generally recommend electrolyte sports drinks, diarrhea is the only symptom that they can actually help. We recommend you discuss sports drinks with your clinician before you try them.

- Try the BRAT diet: bananas, rice (white has less fiber), applesauce (made without the skins), toast.
- Increase potassium-containing foods in your diet—however, we don't recommend that you take potassium supplements or sports drinks containing potassium (i.e., Gatorade) unless specifically instructed to by your clinician. Foods containing potassium include: bananas, apricots without the skin, baked potatoes without the skin, broccoli, halibut, asparagus, saltwater fish, mushrooms.
- Cook a half cup of brown rice in three cups of water for forty-five minutes. Strain the water that remains after draining the rice and drink it. Drink three cups per day. Let someone else eat the rice. We recommend that you stick to eating white rice without the fiber for now.
- Eat bland, low-fiber foods, for example, white chicken without skin, scrambled eggs, crackers, and pasta without sauce.
- It is important to wash your hands after using the bathroom and keep the skin on your bottom clean. We recommend that you use unscented, non-oiled baby wipes to wipe yourself.
- Try lukewarm sitz baths (a sitz bath is a shallow bath in a basin that fits in the toilet seat and is used only for this purpose). Sitz baths are soothing to your bottom and can be taken two to three times a day. Air drying is recommended to reduce friction to your skin, which can increase the irritation.
- Use a moisturizing barrier cream like A+D ointment or a cream with benzocaine to help protect and soothe the skin around your anus.
- If the over-the-counter products you have tried aren't helping provide you with enough comfort, there are stronger numbing agents available by prescription, such as lidocaine.

When You Are Having Active Diarrhea
   Avoid:
   · Foods that make you gassy and increase your abdominal discomfort
   · Fried foods, greasy foods, milk products (except for yogurt, butter-milk, and cottage cheese), bran, raw fruit, raw vegetables, popcorn, beans, nuts, and chocolate. All of these foods can irritate your gut and perpetuate your discomfort and diarrhea.

HERBAL REMEDIES

Chamomile or Peppermint Tea   Drink three cups a day of either tea to ease abdominal cramping and help you to relax. If you also have nausea, we don't recommend using peppermint tea. Since chamomile tea is in the same family as chrysanthemum and rag-weed, if you have an allergy to either of those flowers, you could also react to chamomile.

Green or Blackberry Tea   According to the *Physicians' Desk Reference Guide to Natural Medicines,* green tea and blackberry tea are known to be ef-fective for diarrhea. The tannin in these teas has a tightening effect on the gut and can be very helpful with mild diarrhea. It is not recom-mended that you drink more than five cups of green tea per day.

Nutmeg   Nutmeg decreases the activity in your gut and helps it to slow down. We recommend that you sprinkle a little of this spice on foods as a condiment. Beware—nutmeg has a distinct flavor and does not always agree with every food.

HOMEOPATHY

Arsenicum—good for diarrhea that causes chills, restlessness, or exhaus-tion

Podophyllum—recommended if you have cramping or gas in addition to diarrhea

See also *Relaxation,* p. 252, and *Meditation,* p. 242.

USE WITH CARE

Bismuth-Subsalicylate (Pepto-Bismol)   The salicylate contained in Pepto-Bismol is related to aspirin and can cause stomach irritation and bleeding. Therefore, Pepto-Bismol is not recommended for cancer patients while they are on chemotherapy or abdominal radi-ation treatment.

Psyllium　In the case of diarrhea, we believe the psyllium laxatives (like Metamucil) can *occasionally* come in handy. If you take these fiber products with half the fluid recommended on the label, they can help stop you up a bit. Do not overdo this. We recommend using psyllium this way only once in a while. Do not use psyllium if you are on a low-residue diet. If you are not drinking enough fluid, this remedy can cause constipation.

> *Cigarette smoking is also irritating. Try to quit, or cut back as much as you can. We recommend that you avoid smoky rooms as well.*

For more information on the complementary remedies discussed in this section, see chapter 3.

DIZZINESS

Dizziness is a common symptom of quite a few conditions and medications. For example, it can be a sign of even mild dehydration or anemia, especially if you are also experiencing shortness of breath and a lack of energy (see *Dehydration,* p. 99, *Anemia,* p. 40). Dizziness is also a common side effect of blood pressure or diuretic medications (water pills). Sometimes blood pressure medication will need to be modified while you are on cancer treatment. Or dizziness can merely be the result of jumping up too fast out of a chair or bed. As always, we recommend that you let all your clinicians be aware of all the treatments, medications, vitamins, herbs, and supplements you are on.

> *If your dizziness is sudden and directly related to a change in your body position (from lying to sitting or sitting to standing), be still for a moment to let the dizziness pass. Try to get up more slowly to avoid falling.*

If the dizziness you are experiencing seems unrelated to changes in your body position, or never really goes away except when you are lying down quietly, you simply may not be eating and drinking enough (see *Nutrition,* p. 244, and *Dehydration,* p. 99). If you are having problems with eating and drinking enough, or if you have a fever, see the specific section for a discussion of those issues. If you feel dizzy and just don't feel well all the time, go and see your clinician. It could be that you have an infection coming on (see *Fever*, p. 126, *Infection*, p. 151).

If you are on medication for high blood pressure or heart function and the dizziness is new, call your clinician.

DRY MOUTH

Dry mouth is a frequent problem for people undergoing various types of cancer treatment. It is also a common side effect of many medications people take for other health problems. If you are already taking one of these medications and then you begin certain types of cancer treatments, your mouth may become even more dry. Dry mouth can become more than just a nuisance; it can interfere with eating, sleeping, and drinking, as well as your mood. A dry mouth can also affect your dental health. We recommend that you persevere until you find the remedy that helps alleviate your dry mouth. If your dry mouth is a side effect of a medication, discuss this problem with the clinician who prescribed it. Perhaps you could take something else for the time being.

> *Sometimes a dry mouth is simply a warning that you are not drinking enough fluids.*

Diagnosis and Treatment Considerations

CHEMOTHERAPY

Two chemotherapies that can be responsible for dry mouth are:

- 5-fluorouracil (5-FU)
- Vincristine (Oncovin)

RADIATION

Radiation to the neck, mouth, or other fields around the ear can affect the salivary glands. Whether this side effect is temporary or permanent depends on the total dose of radiation you will be getting to the area. You may notice that your mouth is getting increasingly dry approximately three weeks into your treatments. Very recently, a cytoprotectant called amifostine (Ethyol) was approved by the FDA.

Xerostomia from Head and Neck Radiation   The thick, ropy saliva and constant dry mouth caused by radiation to the mouth and neck is called *xerostomia*. It can be a permanent side effect from high-dose radiation. Xerostomia is not a side effect to ignore. It affects the health of your whole mouth, including your gums and teeth, as well as your diet and nutrition.

MEDICATIONS THAT CAUSE DRY MOUTH

- Opioids—the side effect of a dry mouth is often overlooked when you start on opioids because you are thankful for the decrease in pain
- Antidepressants and sleeping medications
- Antiseizure medications
- Anti-Parkinson's medications
- Anticholinergics
- Blood pressure medications
- Antihistamines
- Medications for psychiatric disorders—prochlorperazine (Compazine), chlorpromazine (Thorazine)—that are also used in cancer symptom management

> *We encourage you to always read the small print of your medication inserts for reports of possible side effects such as dry mouth.*

Prevention

SEE YOUR DENTIST

We recommend that you see your dentist before you begin radiation. Your dentist is an expert on good mouth care and may have excellent suggestions for managing the problems of xerostomia. Your dentist may also want to recommend fluoride replacement therapy or a tooth guard to help protect your teeth during treatment.

TO MINIMIZE DRY MOUTH BEFORE IT HAPPENS

- Keep drinking fluids.
- Quit or cut back on smoking. Smoke is a drying irritant to the delicate tissue lining the mouth, lungs, and digestive tract.
- Check the ingredients of your mouth-care products to see if they include alcohol or peroxide, which can dry your mouth out further. Alcoholic beverages are also drying, as well as being diuretics. Try

rinsing your mouth out with a saline solution. You can make this solution at home by cooking one quart of water with one-quarter teaspoon of salt on the stove, cooling the mixture, and using it to rinse your mouth out as often as you need refreshing.

- If your tongue is getting filmy, make a paste with meat tenderizer and a little water and put it on your tongue. Meat tenderizer is just the enzyme pepsin from papaya seeds and will help take the film off. Many meat tenderizers can taste very salty, so be prepared. If your tongue and mouth are still coated, it is possible that you have too much yeast (candida or thrush) in your system. Have your clinician examine your mouth and discuss antifungal treatment options.

- Stay away from tooth-brightening and dental bleaching products.

- Lubricate your mouth with a little butter or olive oil or a mouth-moisturizing or saliva substitute product such as ORALbalance, Moistir, Mouth Kote (or zinc lozenges). ORALbalance is reported to last the longest, approximately forty-five minutes after application. We also recommend asking your clinician about other prescription products for this problem.

- Use a mild toothpaste, and try brushing your teeth before eating to stimulate your mouth's production of saliva.

- Keep up on your dental care, and ask your dentist whether you need fluoride treatments for your teeth while you are under treatment.

- If you find sucking on hard candies helpful, please use sugar-free varieties to protect your teeth and prevent cavities. Sugar-free popsicles are also good for stimulating saliva.

- Stay away from foods that dry your mouth out, like peanut butter, other nuts, and hot, spicy foods.

- Try eating sour foods, as they can stimulate saliva production.

- Use a lip balm.

- Use a cool humidifier in your home to keep the air you are breathing from adding to your dry mouth problem.

Remedies

CONVENTIONAL REMEDIES

Amifostine (Ethyol)   Amifostine (Ethyol) is an IV chemoprotectant used to prevent damage to the salivary glands from radiation for head and neck cancer. Discuss the possibility of using this agent with your clinician before your treatment begins.

HERBAL REMEDIES

Slippery Elm Lozenges   Slippery elm is derived from the inner bark of the slippery elm tree. Lozenges are the most effective form of this herb and are easily found in health food stores. Sucking on one of these lozenges is soothing to your mouth, sore throat, and upper intestinal tract. According to the FDA, slippery elm is a safe and effective soothing agent (demulcent) for treating sore throats.

SALIVA REPLACEMENT PRODUCTS

It is very important to replace your saliva. There are several saliva replacement products available, for example pilocarpine. Try them to see what you prefer. It is also important to see your dentist regularly, because a lack of saliva can cause dental problems. There is currently a study to see if using pilocarpine before head and neck radiation will prevent or minimize saliva interference. We are waiting to hear the results; but perhaps your clinician can have you enrolled in the study.

VITAMINS

Beta-carotene   One study showed that taking beta-carotene supplements can help with the effects of oral mucositis and dry mouth. It is recommended, however, that you do not take more than 25,000 I.U. of supplemental beta-carotene daily. Beta-carotene is not recommended if you have lung cancer. For a discussion of the use of antioxidants while you are on active cancer treatment, see *Immunity*, p. 233.

WE DO NOT RECOMMEND

- We don't recommend lemon glycerin swabs for the mouth. They are extremely drying and irritating.

For more information on the complementary remedies discussed in this section, see chapter 3.

FATIGUE

Cancer fatigue is more than just feeling tired after a boring lecture or at the end of a work day. People with cancer describe their cancer fatigue as feeling:

- Bone-tired
- Totally exhausted, all the time
- A total lack of energy
- A total lack of motivation
- A total lack of desire to do anything

Cancer fatigue is a very common symptom for cancer patients. According to the Cancer Fatigue Coalition, 76 percent of cancer patients surveyed experienced fatigue with their cancer treatment. Like pain, cancer fatigue is a highly individualized experience. Cancer fatigue is a very important symptom to recognize and deal with early on in your treatment. If you ignore cancer fatigue, you risk major problems with your health and well-being and your tolerance of treatment. For example, if your cancer fatigue prevents you from completing your daily activities, you are more at risk for infection and depression. Cancer fatigue affects not only your ability to participate in physical activities but also your ability to concentrate and focus. (See *Depression*, p. 102, *Infection*, p. 151, and *Immunity*, p. 233.)

Cancer fatigue does not seem to be directly related to anemia or nausea, although both can make your cancer fatigue worse. However, cancer fatigue is probably related to the fact that cancer treatment and healing are hard and time-consuming work. Some cancer survivors report that their cancer fatigue lasted much longer than any other side effect of cancer or treatment. Some cancer survivors even describe permanent changes in their energy level. The Oncology Nursing Society has been studying this phenomenon for years and has led the way in generating the current interest cancer researchers and pharmaceutical companies now have in the problem. There is now active research on possible interventions to help patients better tolerate cancer fatigue.

The most important intervention with cancer fatigue is to recognize it as its own symptom, then try to manage it. Although it may be tempting, don't just lie down and wait until your treatment is over for the cancer fatigue to go away. According to ongoing research on exercise and cancer fatigue, resting too much will increase your feelings of fatigue, not relieve them. Don't give up. There are remedies you can try and ways you can organize your day to manage your energy so that you can accomplish what you need to do, but the first step is to recognize that your fatigue is real.

Diagnosis and Treatment Considerations

Your experience of cancer fatigue will depend on your diagnosis and what kind of treatment you are having. People report that radiation seems to be ultimately more fatiguing than chemotherapy. However, some chemotherapies can trigger substantial cancer fatigue. Bone marrow transplants, stem cell transplants, and major surgeries can have a lasting side effect of cancer fatigue long after the actual procedure was done.

BE FLEXIBLE

Having cancer and undergoing cancer treatment is hard work for you and your body. Even if you are able to maintain your lifestyle during treatment, you may need to make modifications in your daily goals. If you can be flexible with your expectations and goals, you will probably have a less fatiguing time with treatment. We recommend that you listen to your body and do what your body tells you to do. If you need to lie down and rest, go ahead and rest for a little while, but then get up. Unlike other kinds of fatigue, increased rest does not appear to improve cancer fatigue.

> If your cancer fatigue is so overwhelming that you are not able to get up, call your clinician. Sometimes intense cancer fatigue is a sign of infection or dehydration that needs to be treated immediately.

CANCER FATIGUE MANAGEMENT

The first approach to cancer fatigue management is to organize your obligations and prioritize your activities. Start with small, attainable goals. Think about what you really need to do today. Are your expectations in line with what you are really able to take on? During each day, focus on one goal at a time.

First, determine what time of day you feel the most energetic. For most people, this is in the morning or when they first get up. So if you need to lie down after taking your shower in the morning and therefore feel like you have used up valuable energy, postpone your shower until evening, when lying down afterward is relaxing and rewarding. Narrow down the number of things you need to do in a day to the most important. This way, you will feel accomplishment instead of frustration when you review your day.

CONVENTIONAL MEDICATIONS

Epoetin Alfa (Epogen, Procrit)   This medication has been advertised in the media as the answer to cancer fatigue. Epoetin alfa has been approved for prevention of chemotherapy-induced anemia with high-dose cisplatin and is currently under study for use with radiation to prevent anemia. This medication is given as an injection one to three times a week. The injection stings and can be painful, depending on the dose. It also usually takes three to four weeks to know if it will help increase the red blood cell count. For more on this medication, see *Anemia,* p. 40.

EXERCISE

Exercise can help give you more energy, but take it easy. Exercise is supposed to help you feel better, not hurt you. There has been a well-publicized study documenting the positive effects on fatigue and mood of a daily walk for women on treatment for breast cancer. Other studies have shown the physical benefits of even doing housework. Exercise can be cross-country skiing or walking around the block. Do whatever activity you are able to do. It's fine to push yourself a little to get going, but don't push yourself so much that you begin to feel exhausted. You need to find an appropriate activity, given your own individual situation and preferences. If you have recently completed a bone marrow transplant or a cycle of chemotherapy, don't think you can jump up and immediately get back to your marathon training. Remember that even a world-class athlete like Lance Armstrong, who won the Tour de France in 1999 and 2000, had to get back his stamina carefully and with a lot of hard work after cancer treatment. If you are able to walk one block and then a block back, celebrate your accomplishment. Don't focus on what you are unable to do. (See *Exercise,* p. 223, for more suggestions.)

HERBAL REMEDIES

Siberian Ginseng (Eleutheroccoccus Senticocus) Siberian ginseng has been extensively studied as a remedy for stress and fatigue. It is recommended that you take a product with at least 10 percent ginsenosides, the active ingredient. You can buy ginseng in pill or extract form. Buy a reputable brand that contains a standardized ginseng extract containing pure ginseng with no other ingredients, and take 100 milligrams twice a day. Try taking ginseng for two weeks, then taking a week off. Ginseng is not recommended if you have diarrhea, insomnia, high blood pressure, or diabetes, or if you are taking antihypertensive medications, antipsychotic drugs, or digoxin. There is some evidence that ginseng may have estrogenic effects and that it may not be safe for women with a history of breast or endometrial cancer.

Astragalus (Astragalus Membranaceus) This ancient Chinese herbal remedy has been used for thousands of years. Called huang ch'i in Chinese medicine, it is believed to increase the flow of ch'i, the vital life force. Studies suggest that astragalus can enhance immune function and improve fatigue. Astragalus is available in tea, capsule, tablet, and fluid extract form. The typical dosage is one to three 50-milligram pills three times a day or one to two cups of tea a day before meals.

Ashwagandha This traditional Ayurvedic remedy for fatigue has been used in India for three thousand years. It is considered an "adaptogen," that is, a tonic herb that helps the body deal with stress and fatigue. The suggested dosage is 250 milligrams of standardized ashwagandha extract taken twice a day.

PLEASURE

Don't forget that we all need to experience pleasure in our daily lives. How we experience pleasure is a very individual thing. How do you find pleasure? How do you enjoy yourself? Try to incorporate activities that give you pleasure into your everyday life. It will certainly help your mood and your attitude.

RESTING

Although resting is not an effective solution to cancer fatigue, rest is still an important component of your day. When you need to stop and rest, stop and rest. But be sure to limit your rest to short breaks. If you find you need to rest more and more, let your clinician know that your energy level is decreasing and you are resting more frequently.

THE LAST WORD

Cancer fatigue is a real problem. It can be debilitating, and we believe it is even more debilitating to have to endure it alone. Don't ignore or deny your cancer fatigue. Refer to the sections on *Anemia*, p. 40, *Anxiety*, p. 48, *Appetite Problems*, p. 57, *Breathing Problems*, p. 67, *Cancer Pain*, p. 69, *Dehydration*, p. 99, *Depression*, p. 102, *Exercise*, p. 223, *Nutrition*, p. 244, and *Sleep Problems*, p. 192, for more remedies that may help with your cancer fatigue.

For more information on the complementary remedies discussed in this section, see chapter 3.

FEVER

A fever is characterized by your body temperature being elevated above your normal temperature, not due to recent physical activity. It is not known exactly what triggers fever, but it is known that the experience of fever increases your body's need for fuel because fever causes an increase in metabolism. Many people find it difficult to eat and drink when they have a fever, but it is advisable that you try to eat and drink as much water as you can to keep your energy up. Fevers are dehydrating, so if you can't eat or drink, remember that fluids can be soups, juices, or shakes. Forget the old adage about starving a fever. You need to replace the calories and fluid you are losing.

Diagnosis and Treatment Considerations

Cancer can cause problems with the way your body regulates temperature. For example, fever is a classic symptom of leukemia and lymphoma because with these diseases, the body is responding to the proliferation of white cells, which is a common sign of infection. It is not known why fever is common in many other advanced and end-stage cancers, but tumor-related fever tends to react erratically to acetaminophen or other fever-reducing agents.

If you are on active cancer treatment and have a fever and other symptoms such as extreme nausea or vomiting, go to the emergency room. If you are currently on treatment or have an implanted IV access line, such as an implanted port, Hickman, Broviac, or PICC line, and have a fever, call your clinician.

98.6

The average normal human body temperature taken in the mouth is 98.6 degrees Fahrenheit. Some people average a little higher than this, others lower. Body temperature also varies throughout the day. Your coolest body temperature is in the morning, usually immediately after waking up.

An important note for people with cancer is that during treatment, your immune system may not be able to express any sign of distress other than fever because it is overloaded. Therefore, when you feel lousy and your oral temperature is 100.5 or above, you should call your clinician.

How To Take Your Temperature Accurately

There are a few different types of thermometers on the market besides the traditional glass-and-mercury type. It is important that you realize that different types of thermometers work differently and that where you take your temperature is important. Remember that the magic number 98.6 degrees F is for oral temperature taken under the tongue with a closed mouth. Wait ten minutes after eating or drinking anything before you take your oral temperature. It is very important to take your temperature with a closed mouth for accurate results. If you breathe through your mouth, if you are coughing, or if you can't keep your mouth closed for the time required by your thermometer,

Thermometers are specific. Never use a rectal thermometer for the mouth, and vice versa. Glass thermometers have a long track record for accuracy but must be in place for a full five minutes. If you are using an electronic thermometer, be sure the batteries are fresh. Always wash your thermometer with lukewarm water and soap before and after using it— or use the appropriate single-use shields.

use a different method. It is just as valid to take your temperature under your arm (this is the axillary method) or have someone take it rectally. However, taking your temperature rectally is not recommended for anyone with low platelets (thrombocytopenia) or neutropenia or who is getting pelvic or rectal radiation or who has rectal disease. Tell your clinician where the temperature was taken, because different sites have different normal temperatures. For example, a rectal temperature can be up to 1 degree higher than an oral temperature, and an axillary temperature can be up to 1 degree lower than an oral temperature. Electronic thermometers used in the ear are considered unreliable in accuracy and are not recommended.

MEDICATIONS THAT CAUSE FEVER

The biological response modifiers (interferon, interleukin, oprelvekin [Neumega], rituximab [Rituxan], and the chemotherapy levamisole) have fever as a guaranteed side effect. These medications trigger the immune system to produce fever. With these medications, it is recommended that you be given acetaminophen before getting the therapy as a fever-prevention measure. Acetaminophen is frequently prescribed around the clock with these medications.

CHEMOTHERAPIES THAT MAY CAUSE FEVER

- Procarbazine hydrochloride
- Mechlorethamine hydrochloride (Nitrogen Mustard)
- Goserelin acetate (Zoladex)
- Gemcitabine (Gemzar)
- Daunorubicin hydrochloride (Daunoxome)
- Dactinomycin
- Dacarbazine (DTIC)
- Cladrabine (Leustatin)
- Cisplatin (Platinol)
- Bleomycin sulfate
- Thio-tepa

Allergy-related fever is a rare side effect of the following chemotherapies: paclitaxel (Taxol), doxorubicin hydrochloride liposome injection (Doxil), and docetaxel (Taxotere).

Remedies

WHAT TO DO

If you feel lousy or suspect that you have a fever, take your temperature. If you have a temperature above 100.5 (or whatever threshold your clinician wants to be notified about), do not take any medication until you have spoken to your clinician. When your body is experiencing fever, it tries to cool itself down by fluid loss through the skin, so you must drink fluids to replace what you are losing. Dehydration is a very common problem with fever. If you are unable to drink enough fluids for twenty-four hours (see *Dehydration*, p. 99), call your clinician. You may need to get fluid intravenously to prevent dehydration.

> *Dress appropriately for the season and weather. Do not dress lightly to keep your body cool. This approach may backfire and increase your fever. If your fever is high and you have other symptoms such as chills, confusion, or delirium, go straight to the emergency room.*

AROMATHERAPY

Eucalyptus, Lavender, or Peppermint Oil   Any of these essential oils can be used in cool compresses or for sponging down.

Thyme   Spray the room with a few drops of thyme oil mixed in half a cup of water.

USE WITH CARE

Taking a cool bath when you have a fever is okay, but it is not recommended. The fever center in your brain may increase your temperature as a reaction to the cool water. Try to keep your body temperature consistent, not cold or hot.

WE DO NOT RECOMMEND

Alcohol compresses and rubs are not recommended because alcohol is drying and irritating to the skin. Use a cloth dampened with water instead.

HAIR LOSS

Not all chemotherapies cause hair loss, and with those that do, the hair loss is not always total. However, if you are having radiation to the scalp, see the discussion regarding radiation below.

It is true that many chemotherapies, as well as endocrine and nutritional problems, can cause hair loss and thinning. However, this side effect is usually temporary and reversible. What many people commonly report is that the hair that grows back is different from before. Some people report color changes, some report texture changes, and some report both. It is important to remember, however, that the quality and consistency of scalp hair changes throughout your life, and it is not always so easy to tell if the changes are a result of the chemotherapy. If you are on a chemotherapy regimen that causes hair loss, the rule of thumb is that you usually begin to notice hair loss two to three weeks after your first dose of chemotherapy.

> *We highly recommend that you forgo any chemical treatments to your hair while on treatment. This means hold off on permanents, coloring, and heat treatments. This is especially true if you are receiving radiation anywhere on your scalp.*

BE PREPARED

There is no question that the idea of losing your hair is upsetting. But the more prepared you are for this eventuality, the less traumatic it will be if it happens. Be sure to read *Wigs*, p. 267, and consider buying a wig ahead of time while you still have your hair so you can get a good match to your natural hair color. Or, send away for the free catalog of hats, turbans, and accessories from the American Cancer Society. You can find information at their website, www.cancer.org. Some people even use potential hair loss as an excuse to collect and wear interesting hats or scarves.

WHEN DOES HAIR START TO GROW BACK?

Hair grows with its next growth cycle, which can be between chemotherapy treatments. Remember that all hair is not in the same growth cycle. Hair growth cycles last two to three years. Generally, your hair will start to fill in approximately two months after you are finished with the treatment that caused your hair loss. Your hair will return to fullness after approximately one year. Most people report that it takes about two years for hair to return completely to normal. Remember, not all of your hair follicles grow at the same speed. Eyebrows, eyelashes, and pubic hair tend to grow back at a much slower rate than the hair on your head.

Diagnosis and Treatment Considerations

CHEMOTHERAPY

Chemotherapy is often given in combination, so that if each of the chemotherapies you are receiving has a side effect of mild hair loss, you may lose more hair when they are given together. Some chemotherapies are known to cause aggressive hair loss, leaving you with only the hair on your arms.

- *Bleomycin* generally causes thinning of hair. This is rarely total, and occurs three to four weeks after the first dose.
- *Cisplatin (Platinol), ifosfamide (Ifex), and paclitaxel (Taxol)* often cause total hair loss. If you are taking cisplatin on a low dose, hair loss is rare.
- *Cyclophosphamide (Cytoxan)*—some people lose their hair, some people have thinning, while some have no changes. There is usually more hair loss with the intravenous version, but the oral version can also cause hair loss.
- *Cytarabine (ARA-C)*—hair loss is rare.
- *Dacarbazine (DTIC)*—hair loss is a common side effect.
- *Docetaxel (Taxotere)* can cause dramatic thinning but more frequently causes total hair loss.
- *Doxorubicin (Adriamycin)* usually causes total hair loss; it usually starts dramatically right before the second dose.
- *Etoposide (VP 16) and mechlorethamine hydrochloride*—the side effect is thinning hair.
- *5-fluorouracil (5FU)*—hair thinning is more common with high doses or five-day continuous infusions rather than with the weekly dose.
- *Gemcytabine (Gemzar)* usually causes mild hair loss.

- *Idarubicin*—there is usually more hair loss with the oral version of this chemotherapy than the intravenous version. The hair loss starts three weeks after the first dose.
- *Melphalan* causes hair loss in rare cases. Usually there is only a thinning of hair.
- *Methotrexate, teniposide*—hair loss is rare.
- *Mitomycin*—hair loss and thinning hair are common.
- *Tamoxifen (Nolvadex)*—hair loss is rare, although thinning hair occurs more often.
- *Trimetrexate, vincristine (Oncovin)*—hair loss is rare, but if it occurs, it is total.
- *Vinblastine (Velban)*—mild thinning usually occurs.
- *Retinoids* (vitamin A related), used experimentally in head and neck cancers and myelodysplastic syndrome, can cause significant hair loss.

RADIATION

Radiation causes hair loss only where the beam is aimed. Therefore, if you are getting radiation to an area on your chest, you will have permanent hair loss only in that specific area. If you are getting radiation to a specific area on your head, the hair loss will be only at that spot. Be prepared; the areas of baldness can be larger than you expect. After radiation to the head, many people find the skin is too tender to wear a wig resting directly on your scalp, but it is very important to cover your head to protect the delicate skin that is being radiated and to maintain consistent, adequate body temperature. What to cover your head with is a matter of personal preference. Some people opt for a wig, while others prefer a scarf, turban, or hat.

ENDOCRINE PROBLEMS

High- or long-term doses of oral or intravenous adrenocorticoids (cortisone, hydrocortisone, dexamethasone, methyl prednisone, methyl prednisolone, prednisone, prednisilone) can cause significant changes in one's hair quality. The changes can range from dulling hair color, wispiness, brittleness, and thinning to outright hair loss. Some people are more sensitive to these medications than others and will experience more of these side effects. If you are taking these medications intermittently, hair changes are very rare. It is more of a problem for the person who needs these medications long term or as a significant part of a chemotherapy regime.

Remedies

Some people find it helpful to cut their hair short in anticipation of it falling out. With some chemotherapies, the hair loss happens over time; when the hair is shorter, the hair loss is not as noticeable at first. Some people report feeling that their scalps are crawling and unbearably itchy before the hair falls out and have found that shaving the remaining hair off with an electric razor eliminates that sensation. Another good idea is to wear a turban or cap at night so that you don't get hair all over your pillow when you wake up—the hat collects it neatly for you.

> *If you were losing your hair or were bald before the chemotherapy, you may experience an acceleration of hair loss.*

AROMATHERAPY

Carrot, Lavender, Rosemary, and Thyme   In a 1998 study in the *Archives of Dermatology,* aromatherapy oils were shown to be effective in treating hair loss. Essential oils that have been used to treat hair loss include thyme, rosemary, lavender, and carrot. Mix a few drops of any of these oils into a little water or jojoba oil and massage it into your scalp before you go to sleep to stimulate hair growth. We recommend that you try a small amount first to be sure that the oils do not irritate your skin.

CONVENTIONAL MEDICATIONS

Minoxidil (Rogaine)   In a recent study of breast cancer patients, topical minoxidil (Rogaine, used to treat baldness) reduced the time it took hair to grow back after chemotherapy. It is very important to wash your hands after applying this medication to your scalp. In addition, be aware that there can be skin reactions to the salve. If you develop a rash, stop using it. We recommend that you discuss using minoxidil with your clinician before doing so.

HERBAL REMEDIES

Sage and Thyme　Sage and thyme rinses are considered very effective for improving hair quality. Make a tea from the fresh or dried herbs, let it cool off, and use it as a rinse on your hair. Be sure to strain out the leaves. These rinses are also effective in treating dandruff.

KEEP YOUR HEAD COVERED

If you have experienced hair loss or thinning, try to keep your head covered to protect it from the elements. It doesn't matter whether you cover your head with a scarf, cap, hat, or wig. If you are not getting radiation to the head or scalp, it's a good idea to use a gentle moisturizer to protect the skin on your head. Sunscreen application is also an excellent preventive measure, but we strongly advise that you always wear a hat when you are outside.

VITAMINS AND MINERALS

Black Currant Oil or Evening Primrose Oil　For thinning or lifeless hair, supplementing with essential fatty acids may be helpful in improving hair texture. Add either black currant oil or evening primrose oil to your diet (try taking 500 milligrams, twice a day).

WE DO NOT RECOMMEND

Cryotherapy　In this treatment, blood flow to the scalp is slowed by wrapping the head in a cooling blanket or in ice. The theory is that with less blood flow, less chemotherapy comes into contact with the scalp, thus less damage to the hair follicles.

Tourniquet around the Head　Instead of cooling the scalp, a tourniquet is placed around the head to stop blood flow in the area during the chemotherapy infusion.

Why We Don't Recommend These Two Therapies　Chemotherapy is a systemic therapy, meaning that it is supposed to go through your entire body searching out cancer cells that cannot be seen with any test. That is why chemotherapy is infused (dripped in) through the bloodstream or taken orally. If you do something to prevent the chemotherapy from traveling to the scalp, you may be interfering with the overall goal of your chemotherapy.

THE LAST WORD ON HAIR LOSS

Don't despair. If you were not already bald or losing your hair before your chemotherapy, it is extremely rare that hair does not grow back after chemotherapy. As for after radiation, the permanence of your hair loss will depend on your scalp's tolerance of the total dose given. Be patient.

For more information on the complementary remedies discussed in this section, see chapter 3.

HEARTBURN

Heartburn is a burning sensation felt in your chest or esophagus, often after eating certain foods. Heartburn is also, unfortunately, a side effect of quite a few medications that are used with chemotherapy. Despite the name, heartburn is unrelated to the heart itself—the name comes from describing the location of the discomfort in the upper chest and the burning sensation people report when suffering from this problem.

Cancer patients can develop heartburn because of poor appetite and digestive problems, as well as from inactivity. It also can be a direct side effect of radiation that includes the lower esophagus or stomach, as well as of certain chemotherapies. Heartburn can also indicate more severe stomach irritation. If taking an antacid or eating does not relieve your heartburn, you need to discuss this symptom with your clinician. You will probably need to take a stronger prescription medication. Your clinician may even recommend an endoscopic exam to look at your esophagus and/or stomach directly.

Call your clinician immediately if:

- You have gnawing, raw pain
- You are vomiting blood
- You have black stool
- You have vomit with dark blood or with a coffee-ground appearance

Diagnosis and Treatment Considerations

- Ovarian cancer
- Liver cancer

- Colon cancer
- Cervical cancer

These cancers frequently cause fluid to build up in the abdomen, creating pressure on the gastrointestinal system, which can, in turn, trigger hiccups and heartburn (see *Hiccups,* p. 143). If you have any of these cancers, try our remedies, but if you feel no relief, discuss this problem with your clinician.

MEDICATIONS AND OTHER CAUSES OF HEARTBURN

- Paclitaxel (Taxol)
- Aspirin and aspirin-containing medications like Pepto-Bismol, ibuprofen, naproxen, and some oral antibiotics such as tetracycline
- Lying down immediately after eating
- Taking medications on an empty stomach
- Smoking
- Certain foods or beverages (you may notice particular foods bother you more than others)
- Poor appetite or infrequent eating

Adrenocorticoids (Cortisone, Hydrocortisone, Dexamethasone, Methyl Prednisone, Methyl Prednisolone, Prednisone, Prednisilone) The steroid family of medications, especially when taken orally, increase the secretion of hydrochloric acid in the stomach. This increase in acid irritates the protective lining in the esophagus and stomach, causing heartburn and stomach upset. It is possible to minimize this irritation by always taking steroids with food.

Prevention

First of all, ask yourself if you are eating enough. When you don't feel well and find yourself sitting or lying around, your appetite is often negatively affected. Even if you are not active, your body needs fuel to keep your regular bodily functions working effectively. Not eating, unfortunately, makes you feel worse, not better. If your appetite is diminished, try to graze. If you nibble snacks throughout the day, you will probably end up eating more than if you try to sit down to the traditional three meals a day. This type of eating will also keep your stomach working more regularly and may in fact help to prevent heartburn. See *Appetite Problems*, p. 57, *Nutrition*, p. 244, and *Nausea and Vomiting*, p. 170.

CONVENTIONAL MEDICATIONS

Antiulcer Medications You need to be very careful with the new anti-heartburn products that are now available over the counter. When people take cimetidine (Tagamet), famotidine (Pepcid), or ranitidine (Zantac) in commercials, they can eat all the hot, spicy food they want. The reason you need to be careful is because of these medications' potential to interfere with other medications you may be taking. These over-the-counter products can be very helpful if you have bad heartburn that is related to stomach irritation, but you are probably best advised to be monitored by your clinician. You may need a prescription-strength version of one of these over-the-counter products. We do not recommend combining prescription-strength heartburn medications with these new over-the-counter ones.

> *It is always a good idea to read the directions and warnings on any medication before using. It is also a good idea to discuss any over-the-counter medications with your clinician.*

The older over-the-counter products used for heartburn (such as Tums, Mylanta, and Maalox) are generally safe to take in combination with other medications, unless you are watching your calcium or magnesium intake (see *Confusion*, p. 87, *Constipation*, p. 88, *Diarrhea*, p. 109). Always take over-the-counter medications according to the directions on the package unless instructed otherwise by your clinician. Be sure to take the medication when the directions say, that is, before or after eating; otherwise, the medication may not work to its full effect. If you have kidney disease or diarrhea or are on a platinum-based chemotherapy (cisplatin or carboplatin), be careful with all preparations based on magnesium (such as Mylanta or Maalox).

> *If your stomach never feels empty, your heartburn may be occurring because your digestion has slowed down. In this case, you need to discuss this problem with your clinician.*

OTHER HEARTBURN MANAGEMENT SUGGESTIONS

If your heartburn happens after meals or when you are lying down, try to sit up for a couple of hours after eating. If you find you are sensitive to certain foods or drinks, avoid them.

BREATHING

Breathing exercises can often help heartburn by relaxing the muscles around your stomach and esophagus. See *Breathing Problems,* p. 67, and *Relaxation,* p. 252.

HERBAL REMEDIES

Aloe Vera Juice   This remedy can be very soothing to the gastrointestinal tract. Take half a teaspoon before meals. Aloe juice is different from the gel that you get directly from the plant. It is a commercial preparation made from the dried juice of the leaves. The gel from the plant is used externally, while aloe juice can be taken internally. If aloe vera juice causes abdominal pain or diarrhea, stop taking it. It is also recommended to avoid combining aloe vera juice with other laxatives or diuretic medications, such as hydrochlorothiazide (HCTZ), furosemide (Lasix), parsley, dandelion, or nettle.

Ginger   Ginger can help relieve heartburn if the heartburn is not too severe. In studies, ginger has been shown to stimulate the intestines and promote production of digestive juices. Try drinking ginger tea or including some powdered ginger in your food. To make ginger tea, pour boiling water over a small amount of chopped ginger root, steep for a few minutes, strain, and drink.

Teas   Catnip tea, chamomile tea, and mint tea (except peppermint) aid digestion by calming digestive spasms. Mint tea after meals is used for this reason by many cultures.

Gentian   Often an ingredient in bitters, this herb aids digestion by increasing gastric secretions. Gentian is available in powdered form, liquid extract, and tincture (alcohol solution). It is not recommended that you use gentian if you have ulcers. You can take gentian in tea form by boiling one teaspoon of the powdered root in a cup of water for five minutes. Strain and then drink.

Licorice   Licorice is another remedy for heartburn. However, an ingredient in licorice can cause problems in certain people, especially those with high blood pressure or heart problems, or those taking medication for either condition. Therefore, we recommend the deglycyrrhizinated form of licorice known as DGL; it is usually taken several times a day, in the form of a chewable tablet. It still tastes like licorice, so hopefully you will like the flavor. On his website, Dr. Andrew Weil recommends DGL for heartburn because of its ability to "increase the mucous coating of the stomach, making it more resistant to the effects of acid."

Papaya   Eating papaya, especially the seeds, is very helpful for heartburn, as it stimulates the appetite and aids digestion. If you can't find fresh papaya, try chewing papaya tablets or drinking papaya tea.

HOMEOPATHY

Nux Vomica—for heartburn that is worse upon waking.

WE DO NOT RECOMMEND

- If you have heartburn or esophagitis, don't lie down with a full stomach (within one to two hours after meals).
- Avoid carbonated beverages because they distend the stomach with the release of dissolved carbon dioxide, which can be irritating to the gut.
- Avoid eating citrus fruits.
- Peppermint tea is not recommended for heartburn.
- Smoking exacerbates acid production in the stomach, so try to cut back or quit, and avoid smoky rooms.
- Alcohol and caffeine also exacerbate acid production in the stomach.

For more information on the complementary remedies discussed in this section, see chapter 3.

HEMORRHOIDS

A hemorrhoid is a swollen vein at the anus or in the rectum. It is a common problem for most adults whether or not a cancer diagnosis is involved. The symptoms of hemorrhoids are anal itching, pain, and bleeding. Most people discover they have a hemorrhoid by seeing bright red blood on the toilet paper or in the toilet bowl after they have to strain to move their bowels.

Hemorrhoids can occur either inside or outside the anus. They can be painful or not. A hemorrhoid is usually a warning sign that you are straining too hard when you are trying to have a bowel movement and/or your stools are too hard. Hemorrhoids are exacerbated by constipation, diarrhea, and radiation to the lower pelvis, rectum, or anal area. Take care of your hemorrhoid problem early to prevent further discomfort.

Diagnosis and Treatment Considerations

Call your clinician:

- If you see a large amount of blood (more than you have seen before) or red blood and diarrhea together
- If you are on treatment for colon, rectal, or anal cancer and your hemorrhoid is bleeding
- If you have black or dark red stool, are not taking iron supplements, and have not eaten beets recently

RADIATION AND HEMORRHOIDS

If you are getting radiation to an area that includes the anus or rectum, do not apply any cream to the treatment area without your clinicians' knowledge and recommendations. However, a lukewarm sitz bath (see below) taken a few times a day, combined with air drying, can provide you with relief. To air dry your bottom, sit on a toilet seat or lie on your stomach until the area is completely dry.

DIARRHEA AND HEMORRHOIDS

Frequent bowel movements and diarrhea irritate the rectum and anus. Discuss remedies and options regarding diarrhea control with your clinician before treating yourself. However, once again, we recommend a lukewarm sitz bath a few times a day for relief. See *Diarrhea*, p. ooo.

WHAT TO DO

Preventing hemorrhoids is best, but since it is such a common condition, the next best thing is to prevent hemorrhoids from getting worse before you embark on cancer treatment.

Prevention

If you already have a problem with hard, dry stools and/or constipation, use a stool softener, drink more fluids, and eat prunes, more fresh fruit (with their peels), and vegetables if you can. Refer to *Constipation*, p. 88, for other suggestions on constipation management. If you are on a low-residue, low-fiber diet, then you may need a laxative and a stool softener for relief (see *Constipation*, p. 88).

Stop straining. Straining to move your bowels is not good for you. It puts pressure on your heart, head, and rectum! If you are not able to clear your rectum any other way, increase your fluids, modify your diet, and try to remedy your hard stool problem. You may need the aid of glycerin suppositories. See *Constipation*, p. 88, for more specific remedies.

Glycerin Suppositories Glycerin suppositories can be helpful for lubricating your rectum and letting hard stools slide out more easily without straining.

Remedies

TAKING CARE OF A HEMORRHOID

Sitz Bath Try a sitz bath two to three times a day for twenty minutes, or after bowel movements. A sitz bath involves sitting in shallow water. We recommend that you purchase a sitz bath that fits into any toilet seat rather than sitting in a shallow bath in the tub; in a lukewarm bath you will become chilled very quickly. You can also use a plastic basin or a baby bathtub. Some clinicians recommend a cool sitz bath, and some a lukewarm or warm sitz bath, but no one recommends a hot sitz bath. You can try alternating between different water temperatures. See what works for you. An ice-water sitz bath is not generally recommended, as it can be too much for this sensitive area. A sitz bath helps to reduce the swelling at the anus, relieves the burning feeling, and gently cleans the skin.

Creams and Wipes Wipe your bottom gently with hemorrhoid wipes or unscented, nonalcohol baby wipes. Anesthetic hemorrhoid creams and baby diaper creams can be soothing products that can temporarily reduce, soothe, and numb the anal area. The creams also keep the skin folds from rubbing together. Only apply cream to the anal area after drying the skin very thoroughly and carefully. If your radiation field includes this area, do not apply cream four hours prior to your treatment.

CONVENTIONAL MEDICATIONS

Preparation-H Often used to treat hemorrhoids, this remedy is a combination of a yeast culture and shark liver extract. While it is not known exactly how this preparation works, the shark liver extract is believed to shrink hemorrhoidal tissue.

HERBAL REMEDIES

Aloe Aloe juice or aloe gel can also be soothing to hemorrhoids. Apply topically as you would a hemorrhoid cream. You can use the gel of a fresh aloe leaf this way. Many clinicians believe the gel gotten directly from the leaf is the most effective for skin healing.

Witch Hazel This medication can also be used to soothe and shrink hemorrhoids. Soak a cotton pad with witch hazel and leave it on the affected area for five to ten minutes. Be careful when you apply witch hazel, it can sting when you use it.

HOMEOPATHY

Hamamelis—for bleeding hemorrhoids

Aesculus—for when the hemorrhoids don't bleed but there is burning pain in the anus

Try taking two doses a day of these remedies in the 6x or 12x potencies. Stop taking the remedy if your condition improves. Both of these remedies come in an external gel form as well as in pill form. The gel should only be used for up to four days at a time. For more personalized recommendations, please consult a homeopathic practitioner.

LEMON JUICE

An application of a little lemon juice can also be effective as an astringent. Follow the instructions for witch hazel above. Lemon juice can also sting, so be careful.

MORE APPROACHES TO HEMORRHOIDS

There are surgical procedures to remove a problem hemorrhoid. These procedures run the gamut from an injection to create a scar and close off the hemorrhoid to surgery for internal hemorrhoid repair. These recommendations will be made by your clinician should you need more than just symptom management of your hemorrhoid problem.

USE WITH CARE

Because hemorrhoids are such a common problem, there is an enormous market for various products that promise a cure. It is good to remember that since hemorrhoids are veins, astringent preparations that claim to shrink capillaries will probably have no effect on hemorrhoids. Rectal suppositories are designed to be administered above the anus, the area that is most likely causing you problems, but they can be helpful. Anesthetic hemorrhoid creams or ointments will provide short-term relief of painful hemorrhoids but probably will not be as effective in the long term as regular sitz baths.

If your hemorrhoid is not getting better or your bleeding continues, call your clinician.

For more information on the complementary remedies discussed in this section, see chapter 3.

HICCUPS

Hiccups are abrupt contractions of the diaphragm that force the glottis (located at the back of the throat) shut. No one really knows what triggers hiccups. For a healthy person, hiccups are generally a short-lived annoyance. However, when you are ill, hiccups can be more severe and occur more frequently. Severe hiccups can also interfere with all of your basic functions such as eating, drinking, speaking, breathing, and sleeping.

SEVERE HICCUPS

Severe hiccups are hiccups that never really go away, no matter how many times you try to drink from the top of the glass, no matter how long you hold your breath, no matter how many times people try to scare you.

Diagnosis and Treatment Considerations

If you have had abdominal surgery within the past two weeks and now have hiccups, fever, and loss of appetite, call your clinician immediately.

Severe hiccups often occur when you have fluid accumulating in the abdomen (ascites). This problem can also occur when you have abdominal or pelvic cancers or metastases. Your clinician may recommend trying to reduce the fluid in the abdomen (with a procedure called paracentesis), which may be what is irritating the diaphragm or the phrenic nerve and triggering the hiccups. The relief is usually only temporary, however, as the cancer will cause fluid shifts back into the drained area. Be aware that draining abdominal fluid is an invasive procedure and has risks associated with it.

Remedies

CONVENTIONAL MEDICATIONS

Antispasmodic and antipsychotic medications such as chlorpromazine (Thorazine) have been used to manage hiccups but are not always effective. It is important to be aware that these medications also have other side effects and can't be combined with certain other medications you may already be taking. For example, it is not a good idea to mix prochlorperazine (Compazine) with chlorpromazine (Thorazine). Muscle relaxants and antispasmodics such as baclofen are sometimes prescribed for hiccups, but they can also interfere with other medications you may already be taking.

Another approach to this problem is to use medications recommended for heartburn management (see *Heartburn*, p. 135), but this must be done with your clinicians' supervision to prevent drug–drug interactions, even for over-the-counter medications such as cimetidine (Tagamet), ranitidine (Zantac), and famotidine (Pepcid).

HERBAL REMEDIES

Chamomile   Chamomile is reputed to act as an antispasmodic when prepared as warm tea. The component of chamomile believed responsible for this effect is called bisabolol. To ensure that you are getting the active ingredient, buy tea from a reputable source and check to see that it contains the whole flower heads. Drink up to two cups per day. We do not recommend taking chamomile with sedatives or antianxiety medications such as lorazepam (Ativan), alprazolam (Xanax), or herbs used to relieve anxiety such as valerian or kava kava. Also be aware that if you are allergic to ragweed, daisies, chrysanthemums, or yarrow, there is a possibility of an allergic reaction with chamomile.

Dill Seeds   According to *The PDR Family Guide to Natural Medicines* (Three Rivers Press, 1999), dill seeds may relieve spasms, including hiccups. Try making whole dill seeds into a tea.

Lemon Juice   Drinking eight ounces of warm water with the juice of half a lemon is helpful for relaxation. It is not recommended, however, if you have mouth sores.

Peppermint   In addition to being a wonderful flavor for candy, peppermint oil contains menthol, which is soothing to the gastric system and aids digestion. It also has a very pleasant taste. We recommend drinking peppermint tea or taking coated peppermint oil capsules in doses of 0.2–0.4 milliliter a day. Do not ingest pure menthol, as it is poisonous. And do not ingest peppermint if you are allergic to menthol. If you have gallstones, heartburn or acid reflux, it is recommended you avoid peppermint altogether.

HOMEOPATHIC REMEDIES

Ignatia—for diaphragmatic spasms.

For more information on the complementary remedies discussed in this section, see chapter 3.

HOT FLASHES

A hot flash is experienced as a sudden sensation of heat, often around the head and neck. When you have a hot flash, your face may suddenly turn red or your forehead can break out in beads of sweat. Hot flashes can appear and disappear out of the blue, which is what makes them so disconcerting. Hot flashes are also highly individualized; rarely do two people experience them in the same way. No one knows exactly what causes hot flashes, although there are several theories. What is understood so far is that there appears to be a relationship to the changes of hormone lev-

What is also interesting about perimenopausal hot flashes is that they are more prevalent among women living in the West than women living in Japan. Researchers theorize that the low-fat and high-soy content in the average Japanese woman's diet may be what makes her less susceptible to hot flashes.

els (testosterone or estrogen) available in the body and the onset of hot flashes.

Interestingly, both men and women produce estrogen; women just produce more. Certain procedures and medications can also trigger the changes in these hormone levels to bring on hot flashes.

Diagnosis and Treatment Considerations

Cancer and cancer treatment can cause many hormonal changes in the body. For example, tamoxifen and anastrazole (Arimidex) can trigger hot flashes, although they very rarely cause menopause.

Men can experience hot flashes as well, when taking an oral anti-androgen therapy for prostate cancer such as flutamide (Casodex) or estramustine (Emcyt). Other cancer treatments, including radiation to the pelvis and ovaries and chemotherapy with cyclophosphamide (Cytoxan) or busulfan, can bring on early menopause in a premenopausal woman (see *Menopause*, p. 153). A rare temporary side effect of intravenous cyclophosphamide can be facial flushing and a longish hot flash. This side effect can be surprising but usually wears off a few hours after the drug is infused.

Antiandrogens These medications are used to moderate or ablate (prevent the action of) sex hormones when you have a cancer that uses these hormones to grow, such as estrogen receptor positive breast cancer or prostate cancer. Antiandrogens include anastrazole (Arimidex), flutamide (Casodex), tamoxifen (Nolvadex), and citrate raloxifene (Evista).

It has been noted about antiandrogens that the frequency of hot flashes can sometimes be related to the time of day you take your medication. If you take your medication in the morning and proceed to have hot flashes throughout the day, try taking your medication in the evening and see if your hot flashes are less disturbing at night. Many people experience a reduction in hot flashes the longer they are on the medication, which means the hot flashes won't last forever.

If you are a menopausal woman cur-

> *Relaxation and calming visualizations can also be very helpful in managing stress, which can induce hot flashes. See* Meditation, *p. 242,* Relaxation, *p. 252,* Stress, *p. 264.*

rently on hormone replacement therapy, you may have had to stop hormone therapy to receive cancer treatment, bringing back some of the unpleasant symptoms of menopause. We suggest you continue to read this section and see if any of the remedies appeal to you. You can also discuss the problems you are having with your clinician to learn your options.

Cool yourself off by placing cold compresses around your neck for a soothing, cooling sensation when you feel particularly vulnerable to hot flashes. Another technique to try when you feel a hot flash coming on: suck on an ice cube or drink ice water.

Prevention

For some people, it is possible to reduce consumption of food and drinks that can trigger or exacerbate hot flashes. These would include coffee, alcohol, chocolate, sodas, and very sugary and spicy foods. Experiment to see if you are sensitive to any particular food or drink and cut back on it or eliminate it entirely.

LAYER YOUR CLOTHING FOR QUICK FIXES

Dress in layers so that you can peel off clothes or put on clothes depending on your needs. Try dressing in blended natural fibers like cotton, silk, and wool blends. These fabrics can absorb perspiration yet still be warm when they're damp. Linen is also a fabric that breathes very well and is comfortable to wear once you have gotten used to the way it wrinkles. Nylon and polyester tend to keep heat in and are better as outer layers. Turtlenecks and garments with long sleeves are also best as outer layers, so you can add or remove them easily.

Remedies

AROMATHERAPY

Cypress, Clary Sage, and Fennel Oils   Some essential oils to try for hot flashes are cypress, fennel, and clary sage. Use a few drops of one of these oils in your bath, or dilute the oil with a neutral oil (such as almond or evening primrose oil) for use as a body oil. Sage, in tea form, has also been used as a traditional folk remedy for hot flashes. Fennel and sage oils are not recommended while you

Results from a small study done in Sweden show promising results regarding the effect of acupuncture on hot flashes for men with prostate cancer. In this study, men undergoing hormone ablation therapy for prostate cancer also received acupuncture treatments. After ten weeks of acupuncture, the sample group experienced a significant decrease in the number and intensity of hot flashes.

are on active treatment, as they may over-stimulate the endocrine system.

ACUPUNCTURE

In a small study conducted at the Yale University School of Nursing, women given acupuncture experienced relief of their menopausal symptoms, including hot flashes. We recommend you only consult an acupuncturist who is properly licensed. Be sure to let your acupuncturist know about your cancer, and make sure the acupuncturist doesn't place needles in a tumor site. Do not have acupuncture performed if you are neutropenic, have a low white blood cell count or a low platelet count, or have just started on anticoagulation therapy. Make sure that the needles used are new and are used only once. We do not know the safety of acupuncture while on radiation treatment or two days before and after chemotherapy treatment. You may choose to avoid it at these times.

BACH FLOWER REMEDIES

Pomegranate—try it for hot flashes.

CONVENTIONAL MEDICATIONS

The following prescription medications are often used in the management of severe hot flashes, although they have other primary uses.

Clonidine (Catapres)   This medication comes in an oral preparation or a skin patch version. This alpha-blocking blood pressure medication can be helpful, but you need to watch out for signs of low blood pressure (dizziness, shortness of breath, or an unusually low energy level). This medication should not be stopped abruptly. It must be tapered off slowly under the supervision of your clinician. Recent research has shown that alpha blockers may significantly damage cardiac tissue with long-term use.

Megestrol Acetate (Megace)   This medication is a progestin often used for palliation in end-stage breast or endometrial cancers. It is also used to stimulate appetite in those with poor appetite. It can sometimes be helpful for reducing the degree and frequency of hot flashes for people on hormone ablation therapy. Megestrol acetate is not recommended for those on hormone replacement therapy or birth control or with a history of blood clots.

Paroxetine (Paxil)   In a study of breast cancer patients at Georgetown University Medical Center, the antidepressant paroxetine was shown to decrease the number and intensity of hot flashes. The antidepressant effect of paroxetine can also be helpful to lift your mood. Discuss this option with your clinician. Paroxetine cannot be taken with other MAO or SSRI antidepressants—fluoxetine (Prozac), sertraline (Zoloft), fluvoxamine (Luvox)—or sedatives or antianxiety medications such as lorazepam (Ativan) or clonazepam (Xanax) and should not be combined with St. John's wort, valerian, or kava kava.

Venlaxafine (Effexor)   Venlaxafine is another antidepressant that has recently been shown to be helpful with the suppression of hot flashes. Venlaxafine should not be combined with other antidepressants, antianxiety medications, St. John's wort, valerian, or kava kava.

Transdermal Estrogen   There have been a few small studies that show hot flash relief from wearing a transdermal estrogen patch. This patch is not for those with estrogen-sensitive cancers, a history of blood clots, or kidney dysfunction.

HERBAL REMEDIES

Black Cohosh (Remifemin)   This herb, used extensively in Germany, has been shown to be effective in treating premenstrual syndrome and menopausal symptoms, including hot flashes. Black cohosh is believed to exert an effect similar to that of estrogen on a woman's body or on men experiencing hot flashes from hormone ablation therapy for prostate cancer. Although at this time no severe side effects to this herb have been reported, the German Commission E recommends that you use this herbal remedy only for six months. It may also be eight weeks before you feel its effect on your hot flashes. It is recommended that this herb be taken in tincture (liquid) form, in a concentration equal to 40 milligrams a day. Some people have reported stomach upset from this herb. If you experience stomach discomfort, discontinue taking it. It is not recommended that you use black cohosh if you are on a blood thinning drug. Examples of blood thinners are warfarin (Coumadin), heparin, daily aspirin, willow bark, feverfew, and garlic. It is also not recommended that you take black cohosh if you are on oral contraceptives or hormone replacement therapy.

Chaste Tree Berry This herb (Vitex agnus castus), which is believed to work gradually to help balance estrogen and progesterone in the body, is often consumed as a tea or a tincture. The tincture is considered most effective. It can take several months of consistent daily use to realize the benefits of chaste tree berry. It is not known if it is safe to take if you have a history of breast cancer or if you are taking tamoxifen (Nolvadex) or raloxifene (Evista). Chaste tree berry is not recommended if you are taking oral contraceptives or if you are on hormone replacement therapy.

HOMEOPATHY

Belladonna—for sudden, intense hot flashes

Lachesis—for hot flashes that are most intense at night, interrupting sleep

VITAMINS, MINERALS, AND SUPPLEMENTS

Essential Fatty Acids (EFAs) Increase your intake of EFAs. These oils can be found in nuts, seeds, and fatty, oily fish, such as salmon or mackerel. They can also be taken as a supplement in the form of evening primrose oil or flaxseed oil. Evening primrose oil is not recommended if you are taking antiseizure medication; it may interfere with the medication's effectiveness.

Phytoestrogens Phytoestrogens are plant substances found in soy foods and herbs that act like estrogens but exert a much weaker effect on a woman's or man's body. Researchers surmise that these phytoestrogens bind to the receptors that are meant for estrogen, therefore blocking the uptake of estrogen. Cashews, peanuts, oats, corn, wheat, apples, and almonds all contain phytoestrogens, which have been shown to reduce hot flashes. Try adding a few of these items to your diet. Phytoestrogens have not been shown to interfere with the effectiveness of tamoxifen (Nolvadex) or raloxifene (Evista). If you have estrogen-sensitive cancer, however, you should be cautious, as it is not known what the effect large doses of phytoestrogens could have on these cancers.

Soy   We suggest that you eat phytoestrogens in their whole food form, rather than taking protein powders containing soy. For more information on soy (including recipes and nutritional information), visit the U. S. Soyfoods Directory at www.soyfoods.com.

Vitamin E   Vitamin E has been recommended to women with menopausal hot flashes on the basis of the observation that women who were born and live in Asia seem not to suffer from them. Foods high in vitamin E include soybean products such as tofu, miso soup, and soy milk, as well as leafy green vegetables, wheat germ, and nuts. If you decide to supplement your diet with vitamin E, the usual dose is 400–800 I.U. per day. Supplemental vitamin E is not recommended for those with liver function impairment. It is recommended that

> *Vitamin C and B-complex vitamins may also be helpful in reducing hot flashes.*

you take supplemental vitamin E with a full eight-ounce glass of fluid and some food. Supplemental vitamin E is not recommended to be combined with adrenocorticoids (cortisone, hydrocortisone, dexamethasone, methyl prednisone, methyl prednisolone, prednisone, prednisilone).

For more information on the complementary remedies discussed in this section, see chapter 3.

INFECTION

An infection occurs when bacteria or a virus have invaded your body and your immune system is triggered. Examples of common infections include colds, flu, urinary tract infections, and vaginal infections. While you are dealing with your cancer, your immune system is already working overtime, and while you will recover from most infections, prevention is the best medicine. Try to limit your exposure to people with colds, wash your hands often, and don't get too fatigued. Other prevention methods are discussed below.

Despite your best efforts to prevent infection, you may still get one. Don't worry, do the best you can and take care of yourself in order to limit the infection. For ways to limit or manage the symptoms of an infection once you have one, see the section that deals with that particular symptom. (See *Breathing Problems,* p. 67, *Cough,* p. 94, *Diarrhea,* p. 109, *Fever,* p. 126, *Nasal Congestion,* p. 168.)

Diagnosis and Treatment Considerations

It is a good idea to always practice infection prevention measures (see below). However, you need to be extra vigilant with prevention when your counts are down (see *Neutropenia,* p. 178), during your treatment, and up to five weeks after treatment is finished.

SURGERY

If you have had lymph node sampling in the armpit (axillary node dissection), it is recommended that this arm never be used for blood draws, blood pressure, chemotherapy, or venipunctures of any kind. You should also try not to use this arm to lift heavy objects or to do heavy work. Protect this arm from cuts and scrapes, and please don't play with a pet with this arm or hand. If you notice new discomfort in this arm, especially when accompanied by redness, warmth, tenderness, and/or a fever, call your clinician. Even if it has been years since the procedure, call your primary care clinician and report that this is the arm on the side of your axillary dissection.

Edema　If you have edema in your legs as a result of pelvic surgery or radiation, it is recommended that you take very good care of your legs and feet. Always wear shoes that protect your toes, and only use a depilatory cream or electric razor to remove hair on your legs.

Prevention

The behaviors we highly recommend to prevent infection are good hand-washing; avoiding enclosed, crowded spaces for any length of time; avoiding people with colds and sniffles (other than allergies); and not kissing children under the age of ten on the mouth.

- Don't bite your fingernails.
- Discuss any dental work with your oncology clinicians before undertaking it. Take good care of your mouth, meanwhile, by rinsing with a simple saline solution after meals and at bedtime (see *Mouth Sores*, p. 159, or *Dry Mouth*, p. 118).
- Wear shoes and clean socks to protect your feet from cuts or bruises.
- Use deodorant rather than antiperspirant to keep underarm glands unblocked.
- Use sanitary napkins rather than tampons, as they are less invasive.
- Use a condom during sexual intercourse, and be sure to use adequate and appropriate lubricant.
- Use gloves when you are cleaning and washing dishes to protect your hands.
- Use mild soaps to wash your hands and body.
- Always apply sunscreen for at least thirty minutes before going outside, even if you never leave the shadows. A sunburn puts your immune system at risk.
- Don't roughhouse with pets. Don't let birds, cats, dogs, or any other animals bite or scratch you, even playfully, while you are undergoing treatment.

- There is no special need for antibacterial soaps and products. Washing your hands with soap and water with adequate rubbing does the same job, and in addition, kills viruses, which antibacterials cannot do.
- Manicures and pedicures are not recommended while you are on cancer treatment.
- Don't have an enema without first discussing the safety of one for you with your clinician.

MENOPAUSE

Menopause occurs when a woman's body stops producing estrogen (see *Hot Flashes*, p. 145). Typically, this happens to women somewhere between the ages of forty-five and fifty-five. However, surgical removal of the ovaries and certain types of cancer treatment can also trigger premature menopause.

WILL I STILL GET MY PERIOD DURING TREATMENT?

If you are female and not yet postmenopausal, you may still continue to get your menstrual period while on treatment. If your clinicians are worried about the possibility of blood loss and anemia, they may recommend that you take hormones to put your menstrual period on hold for a while. This is very common for young women who will get a bone marrow transplant or women on treatment for leukemia.

SYMPTOMS OF MENOPAUSE

Some women breeze through menopause with few symptoms, while others suffer from a variety of symptoms, including hot flashes (see *Hot Flashes*, p. 145), night sweats, vaginal dryness, weight gain, decreased libido, and mood swings. The difficulty with treatment-induced menopause is the sudden onset of symptoms.

CARDIOVASCULAR CHANGES WITH MENOPAUSE

After a woman has gone through menopause, her body metabolizes cholesterol differently. Up until very recently the belief was that the lack of estrogen decreased the levels of HDL (high-density lipoproteins—the "good cholesterol") and increased the LDL cholesterol. This change in cholesterol metabolism is believed to be at the root of the increased risk of cardiovascular disease with postmenopausal women. Recent studies have concluded that the presence or absence of estrogen (alone or with progesterone) appears to have no significant effect on this problem.

OSTEOPOROSIS

Osteoporosis is a very serious health concern for all women as they age because weak bones are a threat to health and well-being. One question clinicians and researchers are asking is whether taking extra calcium will significantly improve or maintain bone density after menopause. If you are a woman on active treatment for breast cancer or with a history of breast cancer, multiple

> *Calcium citrate is absorbed better than the more common calcium carbonate.*

myeloma, or lung cancer, supplemental calcium is not necessarily safe for you. Discuss with your clinician how much extra calcium is recommended. You may be told that you do not need to take any extra calcium, or you may be advised to limit the amount of calcium you get in your diet.

SKIN AND VAGINAL CHANGES

Because of the loss of estrogen production in your body, over time you may notice changes in the quality of your skin, as it becomes less supple and pliable. A thickened waist is also common. What many women do not consider is that the vaginal mucosa (lining) can also lose its supple pliable quality, and if this is ignored, sexual intercourse and pelvic exams can become painful, if not impossible. If you are not having regular intercourse, please discuss vaginal dilators with a women's health clinician. Vaginal dilators are simple to use and help prevent the estrogen-deprived vaginal tissue from sticking together and collapsing in on itself.

Vaginal dryness and changes in the acid/base balance of the vaginal secretions can also make you more prone to yeast infections and urinary tract infections (UTIs). See *Urination Problems,* p. 206, for remedies for UTIs. As for vaginal dryness, there are a number of good vaginal lubricants and moisturizers available. Replens, Astroglide, and Surgilube are all fine to use, depending on your personal preference. We do not recommend petroleum jelly or any product that is not specifically intended for internal use. We recommend that you use these vaginal lubricants daily, applying with a vaginal applicator or finger.

Disease and Treatment Considerations

SURGERY

Surgical removal of the ovaries will cause menopause. If you are going to have gynecological surgery, discuss surgical menopause with your surgeon.

CHEMOTHERAPY

If you are a premenopausal female and chemotherapy is being discussed as a treatment option, you should ask your clinician specifically about the possibility of menopause. Some chemotherapy treatments can accelerate the process of menopause for women who are in their late thirties.

Women over the age of thirty-five are more likely to go into permanent premature menopause from the alkylating chemotherapies:

Alkylating Agents
- Carmustine (BiCNU, BCNU)
- Cisplatin (Cis-Platinum, CDDP, Platinol)
- Cyclophaosphamide (Cytoxan)
- Dacarbarzine (DTIC—Dome)
- Estamustine phosphate (Estracyte, Emcyt)
- Ifosfamide (IFEX)
- Lomustine (CCNU)
- Mechlorethamine hydrochloride (nitrogen mustard)
- Melphalan
- Streptozocin
- Thiotepa
- Nitrosomes

> *Studies have shown that it is the cumulative dose of chemotherapy that is the culprit in changes in estrogen levels, not whether a particular chemotherapy is given in a high- or low-dose regimen.*

Talk to your clinician if you are concerned about this possibility or if you are interested in more specific information regarding your treatment.

RADIATION

The ovaries are not very resistant to radiation. If your ovaries are in the treatment field, or you receive total body irradiation for allogeneic bone marrow transplantation, you will lose ovarian function.

Remedies

ACUPUNCTURE

Acupuncture has been successfully used to treat symptoms of menopause, including hot flashes, anxiety, and insomnia. We recommend that you make sure you are seeing a licensed acupuncturist and that you be sure to inform the acupuncturist of your cancer status.

CONVENTIONAL MEDICATIONS

Hormone Replacement Therapy For many women, hormone replacement therapy is a way of relieving many of the symptoms and some of the health risks associated with menopause. However, the possibility and degree of correlation between hormone replacement therapy and cancer is a serious possibility that is currently being studied, and you will have to decide for yourself whether this risk is worth it for you. We urge you to discuss this issue frankly with your clinician and determine your personal risk–benefit analysis on the basis of your family history, health risk factors, and medical situation.

Tamoxifen Citrate (Nolvadex) Tamoxifen is a synthetic nonsteroidal compound with hormonelike effects. It works by interfering with the activity of estrogen. It is used as a treatment for patients with advanced breast cancer and is now approved for use for premenopausal women with a high risk of breast cancer and other hormone-positive cancers.

In the recent long-term clinical trial of 13,388 women known as the "Breast Cancer Prevention Trial," women considered at the greatest risk for breast cancer were given tamoxifen and compared to a group given a placebo. While the group receiving tamoxifen did develop fewer cases of invasive breast cancer than statistically expected, there was a slight increase in the statistical occurrence of endometrial cancer, as well as increased incidence of blood clots, in women in the trial using tamoxifen who were over the age of fifty.

Raloxifene (Evista) Raloxifene (Evista) is a selective estrogen-receptor modulator (SERM) similar to tamoxifen citrate. This means that it affects some parts of the body in the same way estrogen does, but not other parts. Some of the side effects of raloxifene are hot flashes and vaginal dryness. So far, raloxifene has only been approved by the FDA for the prevention of osteoporosis. Raloxifene's ability to reduce the risk of breast cancer occurrence in postmenopausal women is currently being studied in a head-to-head comparison to the drug tamoxifen. (This clinical trial is called the STAR trial.)

HERBAL REMEDIES

Black Cohosh (Remifemin) This herb, used extensively in Germany, has been shown to be effective in treating premenstrual syndrome and menopausal symptoms, including hot flashes (see *Hot Flashes*, p. 145).

Black cohosh is believed to exert an effect similar to that of estrogen on a woman's body. Although at this time no severe side effects to this herb have been reported, the German Commission E recommends that you use it only for six months. It can take up to eight weeks before you feel its effect on your hot flashes. It is also recommended that this herb be taken in tincture (liquid) form, in a concentration equal to 40 milligrams a day. Some people have reported stomach upset from this herb. If you experience stomach discomfort, discontinue taking it. It is not recommended that you use black cohosh if you are taking a blood-thinning drug. Examples of blood-thinners are warfarin (Coumadin), heparin, daily aspirin, willow bark, feverfew, and garlic. It is also not recommended that you take black cohosh if you are already taking oral contraceptives or hormone replacement therapy.

Chaste Tree Berry   This herb (Vitex agnus castus), which works gradually to help balance estrogen and progesterone in the body, is often consumed as a tea or a tincture. The tincture is considered most effective. It can take several months of consistent daily use to realize the benefits of chaste tree berry. It is not known if this herb is safe to take if you have a history of breast cancer or if you are taking tamoxifen (Nolvadex) or raloxifene (Evista). Chaste tree berry is not recommended if you are taking oral contraceptives or if you are on hormone replacement therapy.

Wild Yam Cream   Yam cream is sometimes recommended for menopausal problems because wild yams are used in the manufacture of progesterone. However, there is insufficient data to show that yam creams contain progesterone or that the hormone can be absorbed through the skin or vaginal mucosa.

VITAMINS, MINERALS, AND SUPPLEMENTS

Phytoestrogens   Phytoestrogens are plant substances found in soy foods and herbs that act like estrogens but exert a much weaker estrogenic effect on a woman's body than prescription estrogen supplements. Researchers surmise that these phytoestrogens bind to the receptors that are meant for estrogen, therefore blocking the estrogen uptake. Phytoestrogens can be found in peas, lentils, beans, dark leafy greens, nuts, and soy products. The suggested amount of soy you need to eat in order to get an "estrogenic" effect is about six to eight ounces of tofu per day (which contains 60 milligrams of isoflavones, the phytoestrogen found in soy products).

Vitamin E   Vitamin E is currently being studied for its beneficial effect on hot flashes (see *Hot Flashes*, p. 145). If you decide to supplement your diet with vitamin E, the usual dose is 400–800 I.U. per day. Supplemental vitamin E is not recommended for those with liver function impairment. It is recommend that you take supplemental vitamin E with a full eight-ounce glass of fluid and some food. It is not recommended that supplemental vitamin E be combined with adrenocorticoids (cortisone, hydrocortisone, dexamethasone, methyl prednisone, methyl prednisolone, prednisone, prednisilone).

FURTHER RESOURCES

The North American Menopause Society is a good source of information about menopause.

North American Menopause Society
PO Box 94527
Cleveland, OH 44101
(216) 844-8748
www.menopause.org

Another good source of information about menopause and the issues surrounding hormone replacement is *Women's Bodies, Women's Wisdom,* by Christiane Northrup (Bantam, 1998).

Dr. Susan Love, author of *Dr. Susan Love's Breast Book* and *Dr. Susan Love's Hormone Book,* has a website, www.susanlovemd.com, where she discusses the issues surrounding menopause, hormone replacement, and cancer.

Another helpful resource is www.menopauseonline.com.

For more information on the complementary remedies discussed in this section, see chapter 3.

MOUTH SORES

A mouth sore is an inflammation of the lips, lining of the mouth, gums, tongue, or throat. This problem is officially referred to as mucositis—or stomatitis, if limited to the mouth.

Mucositis often begins as a tingling, sensitive feeling in the lips, mouth, or throat. When you have mouth sores, you can look at your mouth in the mirror and it can look fine, with no sore apparent, even when you feel the sensation of something happening. We recommend that you tell your clinician when you first have this sensation. The mucositis may not develop further, but it may increase in severity and become extremely painful, making it difficult for you to eat, drink, breathe, and sleep. More explicit information follows on mouth sores, what predisposes you for this side effect, and what to do to get through it with minimal difficulties.

Mouth sores are very different from cold sores and are treated differently. Cold sores are the manifestation of the herpes virus, and usually manifest as discrete, red, angry-looking areas, whereas mouth sores are usually more diffuse and don't necessarily look inflamed. Both are uncomfortable.

Don't ignore mouth sores. Report discomfort in your mouth and throat to your clinician.

TAKE CARE OF MOUTH SORES

This condition can range from being merely uncomfortable to actually making it impossible for you to swallow, eat, or drink. When people have even mildly bothersome mouth sores, they don't always realize that they are slowly starting to eat and drink less because of the discomfort involved in those activities.

There are some chemotherapies that are pretty much guaranteed to cause mouth sores in everyone. Any radiation to the mouth, neck, throat, or central chest area is likely to cause mouth sores. One thing to keep in mind is that mouth sores often get worse before they get better, but they will get better. In the end, the mouth sores will go away, but we would like you to experience as few complications during treatment as possible.

If you have mouth sores, it is not uncommon for clinicians to recommend pain medication to help you tolerate even mild sores. Your physical comfort is always important, as well as your ability to eat, drink, and maintain your weight. The earlier you let your clinicians know that you are having mouth sore problems, the sooner they can intervene and help you get comfortable. Pain management for mouth sores can run from topical anesthetics, such as over-the-counter benzocaine preparations, to intravenous morphine in the hospital for more continuous pain control.

Diagnosis and Treatment Considerations

HEAD AND NECK, AND ESOPHAGEAL CANCERS

The chemotherapies used for these cancers can include 5-fluorouracil or methotrexate, both of which have a possible side effect of mouth sores. Radiation for both these cancers can also severely limit your ability to eat and drink. With treatment for these cancers, placement of a feeding tube is often recommended. Before treatment starts, the feeding tube is inserted through the wall of the abdomen directly to the stomach in order to bypass the sore mouth, throat, and esophagus. This way, when eating and drinking become too difficult, you will still be able to get nutrients and calories through the feeding tube.

CHEMOTHERAPY

- Bleomycin
- Busulphan—the appearance of mouth sores is usually related to high doses. The mouth sores can be severe. Busulphan also triggers outbreaks of oral herpes (cold sores).
- Carboplatin—mouth sores are rare, but have been reported.
- Cyclophosphamide (Cytoxan), hydroxurea, interleukins—mild mouth sores have been reported, but they are usually manageable with topical anesthetics such as benzocaine or lidocaine.
- Cytarabine (ARA-C)—mouth sores are uncommon, but cytarabine can cause sores at the corners of the mouth.
- Doxorubicin (Adriamycin), mitomycin, dactinomycin, mitoxantrone—with these chemotherapies, mouth sores are usually worse with higher doses.
- 5-fluorouracil (5-FU), methotrexate—when either of these chemotherapies are used to enhance the effectiveness of radiation, mouth sores can be severe. They seem to be worse with the "continuous infusion" type of dosing of 5-fluorouracil.
- Vincristine (Oncovin), vinblastine, etoposide (VP-16)—mouth sores are rare but have been reported.

RADIATION

Radiation is a local treatment, and side effects are usually directly proportional to the total dose of radiation you will be getting. Therefore, anytime you are getting radiation to the lips, tongue, gum, mouth, along the jaw, neck (including the upper spine), or esophagus, you could get mucositis. Ask your clinician if you are at risk for this side effect, and begin to manage your problem with one of the remedies we discuss here. The sores will heal, although it will take time. Your clinician will be monitoring your weight and your ability to eat and drink as a way to keep track of how your mouth sores are affecting you. Don't be afraid to tell your clinician the truth. If you are not able to eat or are noticing changes in what you are able to eat, tell your clinician; don't wait to be asked. See *Swallowing Changes,* p. 197.

ORAL THRUSH

The mouth is an entry point for infection, so keeping your mouth clean is very important. Yeast proliferation in the mouth, called thrush (see below), is very common when your immune system is under stress, as during cancer treatment (see *Immunity,* p. 233, *Neutropenia,* p. 178). Thrush can make eating and drinking difficult.

Prevention

We highly recommend that you try to minimize the potential problem of mouth sores before they start.

- Drink more fluids.
- Stop smoking, or at least continue to cut back.
- Cut out alcoholic beverages.

CLEANING YOUR MOUTH

Don't use alcohol or peroxide in your mouth—ever. Use a salt water rinse after meals and before bed. You can make your own saline solution by adding one-eighth to one-half teaspoon of table salt to one quart of cold water. You can also add one-quarter to one-half teaspoon of baking soda to the solution if you like. Heat this mixture slightly on the stove to melt the salt, cool and store in a jar, and use as needed. It's cheap and easy. You can also buy a sterile saline solution from the local pharmacy, but sterility is not necessary. Please note that a saline mouth rinse will not change the way things taste.

DENTAL CARE

We recommend strongly that you make an appointment to see your dentist as soon as possible after your cancer diagnosis. With your clinician's knowledge, have all your dental work done before you start cancer treatment or during a break from treatment when your blood counts are high and your general health is good. Be sure to inform your dentist of your diagnosis and that you will be undergoing cancer treatment. We do recommend, however, that you wait until after your cancer treatment is done to be aggressive with your gum care. However, if you didn't brush your teeth before, start now. Use the softest toothbrush you can find, and brush gently. You do not want your gums to bleed. The goal here is for your mouth to be clean, not raw. Do not have your teeth bleached while on treatment.

DENTURES

We strongly recommend that you make sure that your dentures fit well before you start treatment. If your dentures irritate your gums, see your dentist for help before your treatment starts. It is possible that your dentures may not fit as well during treatment, and this could affect your ability to maintain good nutritional and caloric intake. Poor fluid intake, dehydration, and dry mouth

> *Clean your dentures well before placing them in your mouth.*

can alter the fit of dentures. Let your clinician know if you are having new problems with the fit of your dentures.

TIPS ON MOUTH CARE WITH MOUTH SORES

- Be careful when eating and drinking hot foods and liquids. Not only is an oral burn or blister an irritation that may interfere with eating, but while you are on treatment, it will take longer to heal. You may find that lukewarm foods and liquids are the easiest to get down. Lukewarm foods also have somewhat less odor.
- Acidic foods can generally make a sore mouth sorer. Bland foods are often the best foods to eat with a sore mouth or throat.
- Brush your tongue with toothpaste to prevent thrush (an overgrowth of yeast; see below).
- Cranberry juice is reported to be helpful with raising the acidity of the mouth and preventing the proliferation of yeast (thrush). If you

can tolerate the acidity of the berries, try drinking cranberry juice on a regular basis.

· Use a humidifier in your home, especially in the rooms where you spend the most time. The humidifier keeps your mucous membranes from drying out. This is especially recommended in arid climates or if you have a forced-air heating system.

· If you need to take medication, know that many medications come in liquid form, which you may find easier to get down. Be sure the liquid medication is not in alcohol, which can exacerbate your sore mouth symptoms.

Is your mouth or throat uncomfortable? Are you able to eat only very small amounts or maybe even not at all because your mouth, throat, or esophagus is too sore? See your clinician as soon as possible. Mouth sores often get worse before they get better, but that does not mean that you have to suffer. See *Cancer Pain*, p. 69, for a discussion of common opioids used to manage pain.

Remedies

Conventional Medications

Maximum Strength Sucrets   Maximum Strength Sucrets are an excellent numbing lozenge, if you don't mind the taste and can suck on a candy. The sucking may also help stimulate saliva production, which serves to refresh and soothe your mouth.

OVER-THE-COUNTER PAIN MEDICATIONS

Benzocaine   Many products that contain benzocaine to numb the mouth are available over the counter. If you are using them for mouth sores, these products should be specialized preparations for the mouth. Most dentists recommend the oral benzocaine preparations for relief of topical mouth discomfort, as they can last a little longer (perhaps fifteen minutes as opposed to ten minutes) and the numbing effects are limited to the mouth. Before eating, apply the cream or gel to the painful area and allow enough time for the numbing action to happen before you start to eat. This numbing action is temporary. We do not recommend swallowing the numbing agent, because you do not want to interfere with the gag reflex. If you have interfered with your gag reflex, you could find yourself coughing when you drink fluids. If you are not sure if your gag reflex has been impaired, sip a small amount of liquid and see what happens. You can use benzocaine products as often as you like, but if you really have a lot of discomfort, we strongly recommend pain medication in liquid form.

Sucralfate (Carafate) Sucralfate, which was commonly prescribed in the past, can help the sore areas in the mouth, throat, and esophagus by coating the area. Sucralfate has also been found to be helpful with cold sores. It must be used at least one-half hour before eating or drinking anything; otherwise what you eat or drink will scrape the coating off. It is usually given in a dosage to be taken four times a day. Sucralfate comes in tablet or liquid form; however, the tablet can be dissolved easily in a small amount of water to make the liquid version.

The "Pink Stuff" You can also ask your clinician to write you a prescription to have your pharmacist prepare a mixture of diphenhydramine (Benadryl) and kaolin (Kaopectate) or Maalox and lidocaine in equal amounts. There are quite a few different versions of this. Don't worry if your clinician writes for a slightly different mixture than is suggested here, as the lidocaine is the numbing agent. Swish this concoction around in your mouth to coat and numb the lining (mucosa). You can also gargle with it and swallow it for sore throat relief, but beware of the gag reflex problem discussed above. Your gag reflex can be numb for about ten minutes after swallowing this mixture. The thicker the fluid, the fewer problems there are with swallowing during this time.

HERBAL REMEDIES

Sage Tea Sage tea can be used as a mouthwash or rinse to soothe mouth sores. It can be made with two teaspoons of fresh sage to one cup of boiling water, or you can buy sage teabags.

Slippery Elm Lozenges This remedy is derived from the inner bark of the slippery elm tree. Lozenges are the most effective form of this herb and are found in health food stores. Sucking on one of these lozenges is soothing to your sore throat and upper intestinal tract. According to the FDA, slippery elm is a safe and effective soothing agent (demulcent) for treating sore throats.

Thyme A thyme mouthwash is soothing to the mouth and throat. Listerine contains thymol, an extract of the thyme plant, which has been used medicinally since the Middle Ages. Thymol seems to have antibacterial and antifungal properties. If you do not want to ingest the alcohol in Listerine, you can make a tea out of dried thyme, strain, and cool, and then use as a mouthwash or drink as a tea.

HOMEOPATHY

Traumeel In a recent clinical trial, the homeopathic combination remedy Traumeel was found to be helpful in the treatment of the discomfort of stomatitis (mouth sores limited to the mouth). The liquid form of Traumeel was used. Traumeel can be purchased in most health food stores.

VITAMINS AND MINERALS

Vitamin E Applying 400 I.U. of liquid vitamin E topically twice per day to mouth sores can help reduce the problem, according to a 1992 research study conducted at the Veteran's Administration Medical Center in Washington, D.C. In this study, patients undergoing chemotherapy treatment for various cancers had statistically significant improvements in their mucositis compared to patients receiving a placebo.

COLD SORES (ORAL HERPES)

If you have had an outbreak of oral herpes, please let your clinician know prior to starting chemotherapy or radiation to your head and neck. If you have never had an outbreak, you may learn now that you have been exposed to the virus. Most of us have been exposed to oral herpes in our lifetime. Once you are infected with the virus, it hides along a nerve until you and your immune system are stressed. Treatment for oral herpes is most effective when you first feel the tingling along the nerve where the virus is hiding. Unfortunately, it is not as effective when the sore is already formed. The treatment for oral herpes is antiviral medications available by prescription.

Remedies for Cold Sores: Melissa Balm You can prepare a strong solution of two to three teaspoons of melissa balm leaves and a half cup of water. Apply this solution with a cotton ball directly to your cold sores several times a day. It may reduce the healing time and delay recurrence.

ORAL THRUSH

Another mouth problem is thrush, which is caused by an overgrowth of yeast. Oral thrush causes a whitish-yellow coating on the tongue and/or the lining of the mouth. Other symptoms of thrush are white spots in your mouth or on your tongue. Thrush occurs when your blood counts are low, your immune system is just not up to par, or your mouth is too alkaline (as opposed to acid). The chemical makeup of the mouth can also change because of changes in your saliva. This problem is also extremely common when on treatment for head and neck cancer (see *Dry Mouth*, p. 118).

Remedies for Thrush   Oral thrush can be treated with antifungals such as *nystatin,* which comes in a liquid form (for swish and spit, or swish and swallow) or troches, which are tablets you suck on. Nystatin is most effective if you allow at least one-half hour before eating or drinking.

Yogurt can help counteract the yeast in your mouth. Whole milk varieties of yogurt tend to have more of the desirable active bacteria. You can also get this active bacteria by taking acidophilus in supplement form.

WE DON'T RECOMMEND

Chlorhexidine or Other Store-Bought Mouthwashes   This is a common antibacterial mouthwash ingredient often prescribed after dental procedures. A large study done by oncology nurses showed that antiseptic mouth rinses are no more effective at keeping your mouth clean and free of mouth sores than plain old salt water (see recipe above). Therefore, we do not recommend most store-bought mouthwashes.

Ice Chips   A study done at the Mayo Clinic found that cooling the mouth with ice chips could prevent or diminish mouth sores caused by weekly injections of 5-fluorouracil. This is still considered a controversial approach, since it is not known if icing the mucosal cells of the mouth interferes with the chemotherapy's systemic effectiveness.

For more information on the complementary remedies discussed in this section, see Chapter 3.

NASAL CONGESTION

Congestion can occur from the tip of your nose to the bottom of your lungs. For congestion involving the throat or chest, see *Cough,* p. 94.

FACTORS THAT LEAD TO NASAL CONGESTION

Nasal congestion can occur for a number of different reasons. The most common culprit is, of course, the common cold. Nasal congestion can also be a result of an allergic reaction or of breathing in hot, dry air, or it can be a side effect of medication. Try to sort out what you believe has caused your nasal congestion in order to find the right remedy.

Diagnosis and Treatment Considerations

SUPPLEMENTAL OXYGEN

If you are suffering from a new problem of nasal congestion and you are currently using supplemental oxygen, call your clinician. This may be a simple problem of needing some moisture in the air you are breathing.

If your nasal congestion came on suddenly and you recently began a new treatment or medication, call your clinician to see if you could be having a reaction. If it turns out that your breathing problem is related to a new medication, see if you can change to a medication that is less of a problem for you. If it begins to interfere with your breathing severely, or you feel your throat swelling, go to the nearest emergency room.

Call your clinician if you are newly congested and:

- You have fever of 100.5 degrees F or higher
- Your white blood cell counts are low (see *Neutropenia,* p. 178)
- You are having more trouble breathing during your regular activities
- You feel pressure in your chest

Prevention

See *Colds*, p. 79, for a discussion of hand-washing and using a daily nasal saline solution.

- Try drinking warm water with lemon juice a few times a day.
- Use only a saline nasal spray—saline helps keep the nasal mucosa (lining) moist and less inflamed.
- Gargle frequently with a saline solution.

If a friend or relative wants to visit and has a cold, ask that the visit be postponed until a day when the person is well and no longer contagious.

Make your own saline solution: put one-eighth to one-half teaspoon salt into a quart of water; cook the mixture on the stove to melt the salt; then cool and keep in a jar for use. Dispense into a clean nasal spray bottle for use.

DRY AIR

Sometimes nasal congestion is simply a reaction to breathing in hot, dry air. If you have forced-air heat in your residence, try a cool mist humidifier. You also need to increase the amount of fluid you drink to help thin out your secretions.

NOSE-BLOWING

The mucosal tissue lining inside your nasal passages is very delicate and tender. We recommend that you only blow your nose gently and use soft tissues. When you blow your nose repeatedly, the skin around your nostrils can quickly become irritated. We encourage you to use a facial moisturizer liberally on your nose to prevent skin breakdown.

Remedies

AROMATHERAPY

Eucalyptus, Ginger, Lemon, or Thyme Oil   Try taking a warm bath with a few drops of eucalyptus, ginger, lemon, or thyme oil in the bath water. Or put a few drops of these essential oils into a bowl of boiling water and inhale the steam. We do not recommend putting a towel over your head over the steam because of the significant risk of burning or irritating your facial skin.

GROSSAN SINUS IRRIGATOR

If you have recurring nasal congestion, we recommend the sinus irrigator, a small device you can attach to a Waterpik. The device helps allow a stream of salt water to flow into one nostril and out the other. For anyone with sinus problems or recurring congestion, it is recommended that nasal irrigation be done daily. For more information about this device and to purchase it, visit the website at www.pharmacy-solutions.com.

USE WITH CARE

Antihistamines and Decongestants   Be careful when taking over-the-counter antihistamines or decongestants, as they can cause dehydration and dry mouth. No matter what type of cancer or treatment you are dealing with, dehydration is not worth risking.

Combination Remedies   We also recommend that you be careful when using commercial cold or flu medicines. These products usually treat multiple symptoms and can prolong your suffering, because the symptoms of your cold are signs and symptoms of your body getting rid of the infection. If you are having trouble sleeping because of congestion, one of these products may be helpful, but try to treat only the symptom that is bothering you. If you feel achy, take your temperature (see *Fever*, p. 126).

WE DON'T RECOMMEND

Nonsaline Nasal Sprays   We don't recommend using nasal sprays other than a simple saline solution. Nasal cold sprays that include more than saline may temporarily clear your nose, but they will most likely prolong your cold by not allowing your body to get rid of the virus.

For more information on the complementary remedies discussed in this section, see chapter 3.

NAUSEA AND VOMITING

We would like to stress the fact that cancer treatment has changed dramatically in the past decade. Almost all of the nausea and vomiting that people experienced in the past is now controlled or even prevented by excellent and readily available antinausea medications. Unfortunately, many people are convinced that if you have cancer, you are going to be not only bald but also violently ill. These days, this is only true in very rare cases. Clinicians who specialize in cancer care know which chemotherapies are potential nauseators and are aggressive in prescribing antinausea regimens.

ANTICIPATORY NAUSEA

If you are sick to your stomach before you even leave your house on the way to your treatment, you have what is called anticipatory nausea, which is best addressed before your treatments start so that you are not predisposed to vomiting during or after treatment. Anticipatory nausea can be managed through relaxation techniques, antianxiety medications, and an understanding and caring clinician. Do not be afraid to tell your clinician that you have this problem. Anticipatory nausea can make you just as sick as eating tainted food. It can also lead to dehydration and poor nutrition just as easily as nonanticipatory nausea. Try eating bland food before treatment. Try nibbling on plain toast, a bagel, or an English muffin—something you are able to keep down. If a particular food looks as though it will make you sick, don't eat it.

> *If you suffer from anticipatory nausea, we recommend that you don't eat your favorite foods. You don't want to forever associate them with this time.*

If you are taking antiemetics and you are still feeling nauseated or are vomiting, call your clinician so that your antiemetic regimen can be modified as soon as possible. Vomiting and nausea are never acceptable side effects. If you are vomiting, you can also become dehydrated very quickly. Dehydration is a serious problem; thus it is recommended that even a little nausea be treated aggressively (see *Dehydration*, p. 99).

> *A "little" nausea is really not an acceptable side effect in cancer care today. Your clinicians want to help you get through treatment with as few side effects as possible.*

ANTIEMETICS (ANTINAUSEA MEDICATIONS)

We strongly recommend that you take the antiemetics your clinician has prescribed. We also recommend that you follow your clinician's instructions on taking them.

A chemotherapy such as doxorubicin (Adriamycin) given in moderate to high doses is guaranteed to be nauseating if an antiemetic is not given at the same time. This is not the time to test your tolerance. If you are a person who does not like to take medications, being prescribed antiemetics may be a challenge for you. But it's worth your comfort to take them.

Whether chemotherapy does or does not make you feel sick has no relation to how well it works on your cancer.

If you have had chemotherapy in the past and had a bad time of it, you may need more aggressive antiemetic therapy than the particular chemotherapy you are getting generally calls for. Like cancer pain, nausea is what you describe, never what your clinician believes you should have.

ACUTE AND DELAYED NAUSEA

Acute nausea is nausea that occurs within twenty-four hours of chemotherapy infusion, while delayed nausea is nausea that occurs after twenty-four hours have passed. Both types can be treated with various combinations of medications, and sometimes it can take a couple of cycles to get the right combination of antiemetics that works well for your nausea.

Think back to what used to work when you were a kid and felt nauseated. These are remedies that always help you to feel cared for. Use the prescription antiemetics recommended, but if your mother always gave you flat ginger ale for a tummy ache, have some of that too.

QUEASINESS

Remember that nausea is not a permanent problem, although sometimes a person can have a low level of queasiness that can linger after treatment. This type of nausea seems to be especially true for patients taking the oral form of cyclophosphamide or a weekly regimin of 5-fluorouracil. If you can be switched to the intravenous version of cyclophosphamide, often the queasiness goes away. If you are on weekly 5-fluorouracil, ask your clinician to keep trying different long-acting antiemetics until you find one that helps you. Sometimes a low daily dose of a corticosteroid such as dexamethasone can be helpful with this chemotherapy regimen.

Diagnosis and Treatment Considerations

It is important to believe that your nausea can be prevented and treated effectively. If you believe that chemotherapy must involve nausea, however, you may have a predictably more difficult experience of therapy.

Nausea can simply be the result of mechanical problems in your gastrointestinal tract. For example, you may have abdominal swelling related to your cancer (see *Swelling,* p. 200) that prevents consistent digestion. Or you may have poor appetite, poor digestion, or other problems (see *Appetite Problems,* p. 57, *Constipation,* p. 88, *Depression,* p. 102, *Diarrhea,* p. 109, *Heartburn,* p. 135, *Nutrition,* p. 244).

CHEMOTHERAPY

The goal while you are on chemotherapy treatment is to prevent nausea and vomiting. Chemotherapy-induced nausea is broken down into three categories: anticipatory, acute, and delayed. Why some chemotherapies cause more nausea than others is not really known. However, it seems related to a combination of mechanical and chemical changes triggered by the chemotherapy. The nausea is not a

> *Trust your body and how you feel. Don't let a clinician tell you that a chemotherapy is not nauseating if you believe it is making you feel sick. The clinician is referring to the statistical information, and you could just be the unlucky person who is more sensitive to that particular chemotherapy.*

> *If you had chemotherapy in the past and experienced nausea and/or vomiting at that time, tell your clinician about your experience before you embark on your next course of chemotherapy. Your body may be sensitized to chemotherapy in general, and your nausea prevention program may need to be more aggressive than it would be for someone who has never had chemotherapy on a similar regimen.*

permanent side effect, but it can make you miserable and can even be potentially life threatening if not controlled.

RADIATION

Radiation treatment fields that include parts of the stomach, lower esophagus, or small intestine can cause nausea and, in rare cases, vomiting, once you reach a certain dose level. With radiation treatments that involve the left upper quadrant of your abdomen, lower chest, or back, a mild nausea can generally start a few days into the treatment, although not everyone has this problem. Try eating a low-residue diet (see *Diarrhea,* p. 109, and *Nutrition,* p. 244) to keep the roughage and bulk in your gut to a minimum while on treatment. Many people have found that nibbling on crackers throughout the day, which prevents the stomach from being empty, can also be helpful. Be sure to keep your clinician up to date with your nausea symptoms while on radiation. If you are vomiting, we recommend that you let your clinician know this before your next treatment.

> *It is important to prevent dehydration! Drink, drink, and then drink some more. Soups, fortified juice drinks, and shakes may be your best bet. You get the most bang for your buck by combining fluid with valuable calories. Drink anything you can get and keep down.*

OPIOIDS

Some people experience some nausea with a new or increasing dose of opioid. Codeine is commonly nauseating and therefore is not recommended for cancer pain management. Morphine can also be nauseating for some people. Often the initial nausea wears off in a few days; in other cases, the opioid may need to be changed. If you suspect that your opioid is the cause of your nausea, discuss the possibility of changing your pain management regimen. See *Cancer Pain,* p. 69, for a more in-depth discussion of this problem.

> *Always take narcotics with food, to avoid nausea.*

Prevention

CONVENTIONAL ANTINAUSEA MEDICATIONS (ANTIEMETICS)

Antiemetics come in various forms, including pills, capsules, intravenous solutions, and rectal suppositories, as well as intravenous injections. We recommend that you always have on hand a rectal suppository version of your antiemetic for when you are nauseated and absolutely cannot take anything by mouth. You may never use the suppository, but you'll be glad to have it available to use if you need it. The rectal suppository usually takes a little longer to work than an oral version (often up to an hour), but don't give up. Some antiemetics come in a sustained release version. The sustained release preparation keeps working over a longer period, which can be helpful at night when you are trying to sleep. Take prescription antiemetics as prescribed and on the schedule recommended to you by your clinician. We feel that it is not worth first "waiting and seeing" to find yourself feeling sick again when it can usually be prevented.

Most antiemetic programs are designed to provide you with the best treatment using combinations of antiemetic medications. The world of chemotherapy changed in the 1980s when an antiemetic called ondanestron (Zofran) hit the market. There are now two more antiemetics in this class. They are wonderfully reliable in preventing chemotherapy-induced nausea for about seventy-two hours after you have gotten your last chemotherapy. However, they do not seem to be all that helpful beyond that time period. Therefore, if you need an antinausea program that covers you beyond the seventy-two hours, be sure that your clinician has provided you with another kind of antiemetic to take for those last couple of days. Unfortunately, these newer oral antiemetics can be very expensive if not covered under your insurance plan.

> *If you run out of antiemetic suppositories, you can make one yourself from combining prochlorperazine (Compazine) with butter or glycerin. Crush the tablet and mix it with a tablespoon of butter or glycerin, shape it into suppository form, and insert it in the rectum. This will not work with the sustained release version, which has a coating—only the regular version.*

MARIJUANA OR THC (MARINOL)

Many people have heard that marijuana is effective for nausea prevention and control. We do not recommend smoking marijuana, as there are definitely health risks to your lungs, esophagus, and mouth related to smoking anything. However, the active ingredient of marijuana, THC, is now available by prescription in the form of a pill, called Marinol. This medication has been found to be more effective when the dose is started low and slowly increased over a week or so to prevent what some people experience as an unpleasant sensation of euphoria. For this reason, THC can be helpful as a preventive antiemetic for the classically delayed nausea predicted with cisplatin. It is also used in combination with other antiemetics and for nausea that nothing else helps prevent. Speak to your clinician about whether THC could help you. It is not recommended for the elderly, as it can cause decreased cognition. Some people do not ever tolerate the euphorialike side effect, no matter how it is dosed.

> *Drinking plain water can be harsh on an empty or sore stomach. Try adding a little fruit juice to the water to dilute it.*

Remedies

ACUPUNCTURE

Acupuncture has been used successfully by many people to treat chemotherapy-induced nausea. We recommend that you only visit an acupuncturist who is properly licensed. Let your acupuncturist know about your cancer, and make sure the acupuncturist doesn't place needles in a tumor site. Do not have acupuncture performed if you have a low white blood cell count or a low platelet count or if you have just started on anticoagulation therapy. Make sure that the needles used are new and are used only once.

> *A recent study published in* Oncology Nursing Forum *discussed the promising results of acupuncture on nausea for breast cancer patients.*

ACUPRESSURE

Acupressure wrist bands have been shown to be surprisingly effective in treating nausea from chemotherapy. There are various types of wrist bands available; some are available over the counter, and some require a prescription. Some wrist bands work by stimulating pressure points, while others emit a low-level electric current. If you would like to try such a device, ask your clinician for a recommendation. One reputable brand is ReliefBand, and you can find additional information at www.reliefband.com. The electrical type of wrist band is not recommended for those with demand-type cardiac pacemakers.

Acupressure treatment for nausea can also be done by pressing a finger on either the center of the inner wrist at the joint or the center of the upper calf just below the knee joint. To learn more about acupressure techniques, see:

Acupressure's Potent Points, by M. R. Gach (Bantam, 1990).
Acupressure Techniques: A Self-Help Guide, by J. Kenyon (Healing Arts Press, 1988).
Acupressure for Health, Vitality, and First Aid, by J. Sandifer (Element, 1997).

EXERCISE

Moderate aerobic exercise can be very helpful in controlling and relieving mild and anticipatory nausea.

HERBAL REMEDIES

Ginger   Ginger is a wonderful remedy for nausea that is caused by a slowed digestive tract. A small amount of ginger taken by mouth can activate peristalsis and help with gastric emptying. Ginger is available in different forms. You can eat candied ginger, drink ginger tea, or take ginger capsules. Some people have found relief by simply keeping a slice of fresh ginger in their mouth during chemotherapy or radiation treatments and chewing on it if they start to feel nauseated. It is not recommend that you take large amounts of ginger if you have a low platelet count. It is also highly advisable not to take ginger two to three days before surgery, because it can interfere in the bleeding and clotting process.

HOMEOPATHY

Ipecacuahna   Try this homeopathic remedy for acute nausea and vomiting every two to eight hours, depending on the intensity of your symptoms. If you have no improvement within twenty-four hours, consider another remedy.

Nux Vomica   This homeopathic remedy is for nausea that feels worse when you wake up. Take the remedy when you feel the nausea.

USE WITH CARE

Aromatherapy   Aromatherapy can be very effective for anticipatory nausea. However, keep in mind that some chemotherapies can cause temporary taste and smell changes, so choose your aromas with care. In a recent study in the *Journal of Advanced Nursing,* inhaling peppermint oil was shown to be effective in treating postoperative nausea. It is not known specifically if this particular aroma will help with cancer treatment–related nausea.

WE DO NOT RECOMMEND

Aspirin or Salicylates   We do not recommend that you take antinausea products that contain aspirin or salicylates (such as Pepto-Bismol). These products have a tendency to irritate the stomach and may very well prolong your nausea. Products containing salicylates can also significantly affect your bleeding and clotting process and should be used with caution. See *Bleeding and Bruising,* p. 61, for more information on this topic. Pepto-Bismol is primarily used for diarrhea management and is quite constipating.

For more information on the complementary remedies discussed in this section, see chapter 3.

NEUTROPENIA

Neutropenia occurs when you don't have enough white blood cells for your immune system to work efficiently. Most of the time while you are on treatment you may have no idea that you are neutropenic until you are told so by your clinician. Neutropenia is temporary, but a low white blood cell count can last longer the more chemotherapy you have or if you have had a bone marrow or stem cell transplant.

Prevention

You are at a greater risk for infection when you are neutropenic. The best infection prevention when you are neutropenic is really the same as any infection-prevention behavior: use good hand-washing techniques; avoid enclosed, crowded spaces; avoid people with colds and sniffles (other than from allergies); and don't kiss children under the age of ten on the mouth or share their food.

When you are neutropenic, it can be difficult to avoid certain problems. For example, common infections such as thrush and herpes (cold sores) can be triggered merely by being neutropenic. For remedies for thrush and herpes, see *Mouth Sores,* p. 159.

OTHER INFECTION-PREVENTION ACTIONS

- Wear shoes and socks to protect your feet from cuts or bruises.
- Use an electric shaver or don't shave at all, to avoid cutting or breaking the skin.
- Do not work on your cuticles or get a manicure or pedicure.
- Don't bite your fingernails.
- Hot showers and baths are not recommended.
- Towel off gently after bathing to preserve your skin.
- Use deodorant rather than antiperspirant to keep your glands unblocked.
- Don't use mascara when you are neutropenic.
- Use sanitary napkins rather than tampons, as they are less invasive.
- When taking your temperature, take it in your mouth or under your arm, not rectally.
- Use a condom during sexual intercourse and be sure to use adequate and appropriate lubricant to prevent irritation or tears in vaginal or rectal tissue (see *Sex and Sexuality,* p. 256).

> *When your white blood cell counts are low, it is highly recommended that you postpone any dental work until your white blood cell counts are back up, usually a few days before your next treatment. In fact, most clinicians recommend that you postpone all dental care until you are done with treatment unless you have a dental problem. Take good care of your mouth, meanwhile, by rinsing after meals and at bedtime with saline solution (see* Mouth Sores, *p. 159, or* Dry Mouth, *p. 118).*

- Don't have enemas.
- Avoid suppositories. If you are currently taking medication suppositories, discuss this with your clinician. If you cannot take medications by mouth, it is possible to get medications prepared for application to the skin (you will need a compounding pharmacist—see *Cancer Pain*, p. 69, for more information on finding and using a compounding pharmacist).
- Use gloves for cleaning and washing dishes. Use mild soaps to wash your hands and body. Intact skin is your first defense against infection.
- Always apply sunscreen at least thirty minutes before going outside—even if you never leave the shadows. A sunburn is a bad idea for you and your immune system at this time.
- It is highly recommended that you only drink fruit juice that has been pasteurized. We recommend that you avoid raw milk and raw milk cheese until your white blood cell count comes back up.
- Change the water in vases of cut flowers daily to prevent growth of fungus and bacteria. A tablespoon of chlorine bleach can also be added to the water. Wear gloves to do this.
- Change the water in your dehumidifier regularly, and clean it according to the instructions. Wear gloves to do this.

Remedies

G-CSF AND FILGRASTIM (NEUPOGEN)

Depending on what kind of chemotherapy you are getting, or how neutropenic your counts are, your clinician may recommend that you use a medication to stimulate and increase your white blood cell counts. The medication will probably be a granulocyte colony–stimulating factor (G-CSF) or filgrastim (Neupogen). This medication is given as a daily subcutaneous injection (into the layer of fat directly under the skin with a very short and tiny needle) for a specific number of days (usually seven to ten) specified by your clinician. Basically, this factor signals your bone marrow to produce more white cells. G-CSF has a very common side effect of bone pain (similar to the achiness experienced with a fever), an effect believed to be caused by marrow stimulation. You can take acetaminophen (Tylenol) for this. The bone pain goes away when the injections are stopped and white blood cell production slows down.

Because G-CSF is a marrow-stimulating factor, it is important to have this injection started within twenty-four to forty-eight hours of your chemotherapy treatment and at approximately the same time every day for as many days as specified by your clinician. Because of insurance reimbursement requirements, you may need to get this injection at your clinician's office. However, it is truly an easy injection to give to yourself. Since you are injecting just under the skin into your fat (very much like the way a diabetic injects insulin) it does not hurt much. Some people report that the injection stings; you can put EMLA cream or another topical numbing agent on the injection site before you inject. Just follow the directions given with the numbing agent you use. Talk to your clinician about the possibility of injecting yourself. If you can do this yourself, you won't have to go to the office or wait for the visiting nurse to come to your home.

See *Infection*, p. 151; *Immunity*, p. 233, for ways to assist your immune system and its effectiveness; *Nutrition*, p. 244, for ideas on how to feed your body; and *Dehydration*, p. 99, for tips on how to drink enough fluid.

For more information on the complementary remedies discussed in this section, see chapter 3.

NUMBNESS AND TINGLING

Paresthesis is the term for the sensations of tingling and burning or pins and needles. *Neuropathy* is the term for the sensation of numbness. Most people experience these feelings as a result of the blood supply to an area getting cut off for a brief period of time. However, for certain people, these sensations don't go away during and after treatment. The feelings can linger for three to six months after treatment is finished or, in some cases, even longer.

Numbness and tingling are symptoms that you need to tell your clinician about. In this chapter, we will describe some treatments that are available if this numbness is causing you pain. We will also give you safety guidelines to follow.

NERVE PAIN

Nerve pain is frequently inadequately treated. It is often described as a numb and tingly sensation or burning, like constant pins and needles. It can be severe. Discuss this type of pain with your clinician for appropriate medication advice. Medications commonly used to treat seizures, such as gabapentin (Neurontin), carbamazepine (Tegretol), and clonazepam (Klonopin), and the tricyclic antidepressants, such as nortriptyline hydrochloride (Pamelor) and desipramine hydrochloride (Norpramin), are helpful with nerve pain, along with opioids. Amitriptyline hydrochloride (Elavil) tends to have more side effects but can also be used. Be aware that these medications need to be dosed at different doses than when dosed for seizure or depression.

Disease and Treatment Considerations

If you have had breast cancer, prostate cancer, lung cancer, renal cell cancer, multiple myeloma, leukemia, sarcoma, or Paget's disease and are experiencing numbness and/or tingling that involves your back, arm, legs, fingers, or toes, call your clinician immediately.

DIABETES

Diabetics can have a more difficult time with tingling and numbness from cancer treatment. See your diabetes clinician to discuss your risk before starting cancer treatment.

LUNG CANCER

While some lung cancers are discovered because of symptoms of numbness and tingling, this is extremely rare. If this has happened to you, the treatment for the cancer will also be the treatment for the nerve problem.

SURGERY

Axillary (underarm) lymph node dissection (frequently done during breast cancer surgery), retroperitoneal lymph node dissection (frequently done for pelvic and abdominal cancers), and other node dissection surgery can inadvertently disturb nerves. For example, lymph node dissection in the axillary region can trigger numbness, tingling, and even pain in that arm. The abdominal node dissection can affect the leg and interfere with walking.

CHEMOTHERAPY

Chemotherapies that can cause numbness and tingling, even some months after you have completed treatment, are paclitaxel (Taxol), carboplatin, etoposide (VP16), teniposide, vincristine (Oncovin), vendesine, and interferon alpha-2A (Inferon).

Safety Considerations   Not everyone who gets the chemotherapies listed above has problems with numbness, tingling, or other neuropathies. However, the problem does seem to be dose-related, and the numbness can begin to happen without you even being aware of it. You may not notice your manual dexterity is impeded until one day when you have difficulty picking up change or a pen off a counter.

If you are getting any of the chemotherapies listed above, always:

- Wear gloves and socks in cool weather
- Test the water in your bath or shower with your elbow or knee, to avoid burns; the joints may sense heat and cold more reliably than your hands and feet
- Be careful with hot foods and drinks so you don't burn your mouth

RADIATION

If you feel tingling in a radiation treatment field, bring this to the attention of your clinician. This is frequently an early warning of a skin reaction. See *Skin Care and Wounds,* p. 185.

Remedies

CONVENTIONAL MEDICATIONS

If you have what we call neuropathic pain syndrome, that is, a burning pain with tingling and/or numbness, you may be treated with tricyclic antidepressants—such as nortriptyline, amitriptyline (Elavil), or desipramine. Or you may be treated with seizure medications—such as Neurontin (gabapentin)—or a combination of tricyclics and seizure medication. These medications can be extremely helpful for neuropathic pain. Be aware that they may take a few weeks to start working and can have their own set of side effects. For example, tricyclic anti-depressants are famous for causing dry mouth. Another intravenous medication amifostine (Ethyol) has been reported to prevent some neuropathy if given before paclitaxel (Taxol).

Lidocaine Patch   The lidocaine patch is an anaesthetic that was developed for managing the nerve pain of shingles. It may help with nerve pain that is superficial, rather than deep.

HERBAL REMEDIES

Capsaicin Cream   Capsaicin cream, which is made with the active ingredient found in chili peppers, works by stimulating nerve sensors for pain in the area where the cream is administered. The idea is that the pain threshold is overwhelmed by this process, rendering the area treated less sensitive to stimulation. The cream can burn, so keep it away from your eyes and wash your hands thoroughly after using. You may wish to use gloves to protect the skin on your hands when you apply it. Different people have different reactions to capsaicin. To avoid a burning feeling, you can numb the area you will treat with a benzocaine preparation (commonly found in teething creams). After applying the numbing cream, wait five to ten minutes before you rub on the capsaicin cream. The numbing cream only affects the surface of the skin, so the capsaicin cream should still be effective. Do not use capsaicin cream on surgical scars that are less than six months old and do not take capsaicin internally.

HOMEOPATHY

Hypericum is often used for nerve pain.

NERVE BLOCKS

In some cases, you can have the nerve blocked altogether. This is usually not a permanent fix, unfortunately, and is best only for short-term relief. A nerve block is done by an anesthesiologist. If nothing else has helped you, discuss this option with your clinician.

TENS (TRANSCUTANEOUS ELECTRIC NERVE STIMULATION)

A pain management device called a TENS unit, available from pain specialists, physical therapists, and chiropractors, has been found to be helpful for nerve pain. This device works by electrical stimulation of a nerve path, elevating your pain threshold and promoting muscle relaxation. Don't use this device without the recommendation and supervision of a clinician. TENS units are frequently used to treat phantom limb syndrome after amputation.

USE WITH CARE

Compresses   Try applying heat or cold compresses to the affected area. Generally, warmth is relaxing, and cold packs are stimulating. Many hydrotherapists use alternating warm and cold compresses to speed healing. If you have numbness in an area, hot and cold compresses can be problematic, as you may not be able to sense if the compress is too hot or too cold. We recommend you test the temperature of the compress with a knee or an elbow before applying. Compresses are not recommended on areas in a current radiation field.

For more information on the complementary remedies discussed in this section, see chapter 3.

SKIN CARE AND WOUNDS

Cancer treatment can cause temporary skin changes and can delay the healing of wounds. If you cut or scratch yourself while you are undergoing treatment, you will notice slower healing. It is best to avoid injuries and protect your skin while you are on treatment.

Some people find that their skin is dryer while on cancer treatment. This may be true for a variety of reasons. You may not be eating the same diet as before you were on treatment, you may not be drinking enough fluid, or you may be spending more time indoors or in dryer air. Dry skin is a complicated problem, but you can certainly try to manage it with some of the remedies we discuss at the end of this section.

Diagnosis and Treatment Considerations

SURGICAL WOUNDS

Surgical wounds are wounds resulting from surgery. It is important that you eat and drink well to help your skin repair and your wounds heal. You especially need vitamin C. This vitamin is best absorbed from fresh fruits and vegetables, which will give you the additional benefit of other nutrients as well. Protein and fluid are also needed for repair and healing. See *Nutrition,* p. 244, for more eating tips.

WOUND SPECIALISTS

There are many, many wound care products for all types of different healing goals. For the correct products and care, be sure to get recommendations from a wound specialist, who is usually a highly specialized and experienced nurse who will teach you and your caregivers how to clean and dress a wound to allow for the best healing possible. Be sure that the nurse helping you knows about your cancer and any limitations you might have. For instance, if you are having a tough time eating fresh fruits and vegetables, be sure to let the nurse know. If the wound is in a difficult place on your body to take care of, you must tell your clinician. You will need help with cleaning and dressing this wound. You may even need help figuring out how to sleep at night with it. Don't be afraid to ask for help.

> *Some chemotherapies also can cause a general darkening of skin or veins. This is particularly noticeable with intravenous 5-fluorouracil (5-FU). This darkening is sometimes temporary.*

CHEMOTHERAPY

Cyclophosphamide (Cytoxan)   Cyclophosphamide sometimes can cause a facial rash, especially with the oral version.

RADIATION

Radiation Recall   Many chemotherapies, other medications, and radiation treatment make you more sun sensitive while you are on treatment. A phenomenon called radiation recall can also occur: This is when an area of skin that was in the radiation treatment field (even years ago) turns darker than the surrounding skin. This can be triggered by medication, chemotherapy, radiation, or sun exposure. Skin exposed to radiation treatment will be more sun sensitive for the rest of your life. Remember to cover this previously radiated area and prevent its exposure to the sun as much as possible.

Radiation Skin Reactions   Radiation sometimes can trigger significant skin reactions, depending on what part of the body is being treated, the type of skin you have, whether you have a fair or olive complexion, and your nutritional health, as well as other health factors. People getting radiation are monitored closely for skin reactions because it is important that your skin remain relatively unscathed while on radiation treatment. If the skin within the radiation field is feeling tingly and sore, be sure to report this sensation to your clinicians for their care recommendations. A tingly, sore feeling in the skin is often a warning sign of skin reaction.

Generally, any skin in a radiation field should be washed as infrequently as possible. You should not rub or scrub the area with soap or even the softest cloth. You can rinse off the area with water. It is recommended that you only use your hands to wash your skin, as they will be the gentlest. Air drying the skin is also highly recommended. You can use a blow dryer only if it has a "No Heat" option. Otherwise you should avoid unnecessary friction and heat when caring for skin in the radiation field. Try not to touch the skin in that area at all. In addition, keep the area unclothed as often as possible, and wear loose, unrestrictive clothing.

MALIGNANT CUTANEOUS WOUNDS

Malignant cutaneous wounds are wounds caused by metastatic tumor involvement of the skin. The most commonly found cutaneous metastases are with breast and lung cancer. If you have this type of wound, see your clinician for proper diagnosis and care.

RASHES

Rashes can be caused by skin irritation or an allergic reaction, and the cause can sometimes be determined by defining the rash. What kind of rash is this? Is it in one area, or all over? Is it red? Itchy? Did you just start on a new medication or antibiotic? Have you recently changed laundry detergent, soap, cream, or moisturizer? We recommend that you discuss any new rash with your clinician, especially if you have recently started on a new medication.

> *Many skin conditions can be exacerbated by stress. See* Stress, *p. 264,* Relaxation, *p. 252, and* Meditation, *p. 242, for ideas on stress reduction activities.*

Prevention

> For general skin health, wear gloves to protect your hands when washing dishes, cleaning up, and gardening. Of course, after removing your gloves, you should wash your hands.

Skin and wound care is very much a matter of common sense. There is no difference between how you should treat your skin and wounds when you have cancer and how you should treat them when you don't. Simply wash wounds daily with mild soap and water and dry carefully. Always towel off gently. A bracing rubdown is best avoided while on treatment.

SKIN CARE

We recommend that you always use a mild soap to wash yourself. If you use a commercial moisturizing cream, we recommend that you read the

> Always apply moisturizer to wet skin. This will increase the moisturizing effect.

ingredients and make sure that mineral oil and alcohol (in any form) are not listed as ingredients. Some moisturizers seem to moisturize but ultimately dry out your skin. The product with the shortest list of ingredients is usually the safest to use. Simpler is better. Fragrances can also cause skin problems, so we recommend that you choose an unscented product if possible.

WOUND CARE

Always wash your hands before taking care of a wound. Wash your hands before you remove the old dressing and then again before you redress it. No wound is sterile, but wound care should be as clean

> Make your own saline solution by heating one quart of water with one-eighth to one-half teaspoon of salt; warm until salt dissolves, let cool, and use.

as possible. Some wounds do not need to be cleaned with soap and water and can be rinsed off gently with saline solution.

If you have a wound that is raw or oozing, gently clean it first with mild soap and lukewarm water, then gently cover it with loose gauze. Otherwise, leave the wound uncovered to let it get air.

SHOWERS VERSUS BATHS

To protect your skin, taking showers is usually recommended over soaking in baths. Long, hot showers and baths are drying to the skin. That is why there are so many moisturizing bath products. To rest your skin, we recommend that you try not to bathe every day. While there is no denying the pleasures of a relaxing soak in the bathtub, you should take long soaking baths less often.

Some commercial bath products, especially bubble baths, can be irritating to your skin. Read the ingredients to try to find a more organic product, or instead add a few drops of almond oil and some dry milk to your bath for a moisturizing effect.

SUN SENSITIVITY

It should probably go without saying that we do not recommend tanning or sun exposure for anyone, regardless of cancer history. We would like to point out, however, that the bulk of unprotected sun exposure most people get occurs during the walk from car to home or office. So, although we recommend against lying out in the sun, we also recommend always wearing and reapplying sunscreen on skin that is exposed to air. It is generally a good idea to limit your exposure to direct sunlight and take care to apply sunscreen with an SPF of fifteen to thirty strength a few times a day to any exposed skin. Don't forget to apply it to your ears, the back of your neck, and the back of your hands, as well as your face.

Remedies

AROMATHERAPY

Chamomile, Lavender, and Sandalwood oil   To make a moisturizing oil to apply to the body, mix four drops of up to three different essential oils in two tablespoons of a base oil. For dry skin, we recommend chamomile, lavender, or sandalwood.

LAVENDER

Lavender is one of the most popular essential oils. It can be used for burns, insect bites, and minor cuts. Before applying, dilute lavender with a base oil such as wheat germ, almond, or evening primrose oil.

CUCUMBER

Cucumber is known to be soothing and cooling to the skin. We recommend you take slices of cucumber and lay them flat on the irritated area, rather than buying a commercial cucumber cream. Fresh cucumber is quite safe to use on skin, even radiated skin. Cucumber can also be soothing for an itchy rash.

GIRDLES

After surgery, the affected area can feel sore, and, depending on the location of the surgery, your activities can become limited. If your surgical wound is in your pelvis or abdomen, wearing a girdle can help support your abdomen during healing and help you move about more comfortably.

HERBAL REMEDIES

Aloe Gel   The aloe gel that you can get from peeling the leaf of a house plant is very cooling and soothing to irritated or sore skin. You can also buy pure aloe gel in a health food store or drugstore. Aloe gel is safe to use on radiated skin, but it is not recommended for use for four hours before your treatment. Do not use aloe if you are sensitive or allergic to latex.

Calendula   Calendula flowers have long been used as a remedy for skin irritations, burns, bruises, and rashes. You can buy calendula creams and ointments, or you can make calendula tea by pouring one cup of boiling water over one to two teaspoons of calendula flowers. When cooled, this tea can be used topically on the skin. Homeopathic calendula ointments are also used externally for burns.

Chamomile   Chamomile flowers have traditionally been used both internally and externally. Externally, in a compress, chamomile can help with minor skin irritations. To make a chamomile compress, pour one cup of hot water over two teaspoons of chamomile flowers or a chamomile teabag. Cover, steep, and then strain. Soak a cloth in the warm water and apply it to the affected area a few times a day. If you are allergic to chrysanthemums, daises, ragweed, or yarrow, we don't recommend using chamomile, as it may cause a similar allergic reaction.

Goldenseal   This traditional herb (*hydrastis canadensis L.*), used by the Cherokee Indians, has been used as a skin wash. The herb seems to affect the mucous membranes by drying up secretions, reducing inflammation, and fighting infection through the mild antimicrobial action of its active ingredient, berberine. You can buy goldenseal as a tincture (liquid) or in tea form. Try applying goldenseal in a compress, or apply a few drops directly to the affected area.

Gotu Kola   An Ayurvedic herb, gotu kola (*centulla asiatica*) has traditionally been used for wound healing and chronic skin conditions, including leprosy, as well as eczema and psoriasis. Taken internally, it is believed to speed the healing of wounds. Applied topically, it seems to help the healing of scars. You can make a compress using one-half teaspoon of the herb to one cup of water. You can also find gotu kola in tincture or extract form. The generally recommended dose for taking gotu kola internally in a tincture is 10 to 20 milliliters a day.

St. John's Wort   Although St. John's wort is generally used as an internal remedy for depression, it is also used externally to reduce inflammation and promote healing, because of its antibacterial properties. We recommend you use a few drops of St. John's wort oil on the irritated area; discontinue if any irritation develops. Be aware that St. John's wort oil is red and may stain clothing.

Tea Tree Oil   Found in Australia, tea tree oil is contained in many products, including toothpaste, mouth rinses, and shampoos. Tea tree oil is believed to have significant antimicrobial and antifungal properties. We recommend that you always dilute tea tree oil with a little water or oil before applying it directly to the skin. It is not recommended that you apply tea tree oil to skin in a radiation field or to open or blistered skin.

OATMEAL BATHS

This remedy may appear to be a contradiction, but oatmeal can be very soothing to the skin. For extremely dry and irritated skin, try an oatmeal bath product, following the directions on the package.

TEA BAGS

Moistened tea bags can give relief to cracked, irritated, dry skin. Lay the cool, wet tea bag on the irritated area for relief. Use regular black tea; it is the tannins in the tea that are helpful here. We do not recommend using wet tea bags on open or blistered wounds.

VITAMINS AND MINERALS

Vitamin E   Vitamin E oil can be applied directly to a closed wound or incision to help prevent scar buildup. It is very important that the wound is entirely closed before you apply it. You can use a vitamin E capsule; squeeze the contents onto your skin and gently massage it in.

WE DO NOT RECOMMEND

Creams and Salves   Using creams and salves on a wound is generally not recommended unless prescribed by your clinician. If the wound is not clean and dry, the cream or salve can actually lock in bacteria and dirt and further infect the wound. The most important way to prevent infection is washing the wound area daily and gently with soap and water and air drying it.

Peroxide and Iodine   Save the peroxide for your teeth or for denture cleaning. We also do not recommend iodine or iodine-containing washes or creams. Peroxide, iodine, and similar products all break down your body's own healing processes. With deep or very dirty wounds, it is recommended that you see your clinician or go to the emergency room.

For more information on the complementary remedies discussed in this section, see chapter 3.

SLEEP PROBLEMS

Everyone experiences problems with sleep from time to time. However, if this is a frequent problem for you and you are not feeling rested after sleep, it is important that you address this problem. Sleep serves many vital functions besides providing rest. The deep stage IV sleep helps your body to do the work of healing and repair and allows your immune system to function more effectively. Even your dreams help you to mentally process all the events of your day and life.

IS IT INSOMNIA?

Some typical symptoms of insomnia are:

- You lie in bed but can't get to sleep.
- You wake up in the middle of the night and can't go back to sleep.
- You wake up very early in the morning and you can't get back to sleep.

If you have any of these symptoms for more than a couple of days, you are experiencing insomnia.

SOURCES OF SLEEP PROBLEMS

Think about what's going on in your life and try to direct your attention to the underlying problem that may be interfering with your sleep. Insomnia can be caused by a variety of things, including breathing problems, appetite problems, depression, anxiety, fatigue, or nutrition. Refer to the relevant sections for more suggestions on how to cope with these issues.

Many medications have side effects that can disrupt your sleep. See below for more on medications and sleep.

Insomnia, depression, and anxiety can become a vicious cycle. If you are depressed, you won't sleep as deeply. When you have less deep sleep, you feel more anxious. If you feel anxious, you will sleep less. Try to deal with the problems that interfere with your sleep as soon as they occur to prevent this endless cycle.

NOT ALL SLEEP IS EQUAL

The different phases of sleep provide your body with different benefits. Therefore, if sleeping at night is a problem for you, napping frequently during the day is not necessarily the way to catch up on sleep. Napping is fine, but you still have to deal with the underlying problem that is disrupting your sleep. Research shows that meditation and relaxation exercises can provide some of the effects of deep sleep if done regularly. Practicing meditation and relaxation exercises will also improve the quality of your sleep by helping to relieve stress and relax you.

Diagnosis and Treatment Considerations

MEDICATIONS

If you suspect that your problems with sleep started with the addition or increase of a dose of medication, read the information provided with the medication and see if sleep problems are listed as one of the reported side effects. Even if sleep problems are not indicated, adrenocorticoids, opioids, stimulants (including caffeine), and blood pressure medications can all interfere with the quality of your sleep.

Oddly enough, the prescription sleep aids that are meant to help you with your sleep can prevent your sleep from advancing through all the different phases. These medications are fine for occasional use but will not solve the problem of insomnia. After using these sedating medications, people often complain about waking up feeling dried up and groggy, which can interfere with the quality of your awake time. Therefore, we believe that prescription sleep aids are best used on a temporary basis.

Sleeping Pills and Other Prescription Sleep Aids   For the occasional problem getting to sleep, it is probably fine to use either over-the-counter or prescription sleep aids such as antihistamines or sedatives. However, the problem with long-term use of sleep aids is that they don't usually improve your sleep for more than a few nights. In addition, as we discussed, the sleep that you do get is not always restorative.

PAIN

Pain can seriously affect the quality of your sleep even if it does not prevent you from sleeping. Opioids prescribed for pain can also interfere with sleep. It is important to manage the pain, however, so it does not cause other problems that can interfere with your sleep, such as depression, inactivity, discomfort, and despair. You must consider the risks versus the benefits of opioids in this case. If the benefits outweigh the risks for you, then the medication is probably worthwhile.

Prevention

One of the most important ways to prevent insomnia is by keeping regular sleep habits.

- Go to bed only when sleepy.
- Avoid caffeine, nicotine, and alcohol for four to six hours before you go to sleep. We advise that you avoid nicotine altogether.
- Use the bed only for sleeping. This way you will associate your bed only with sleep.
- Try not to work, watch television, read, or eat in bed.
- Set the alarm for the same time every morning, and get up when it goes off.
- Keep the bedroom cool, dark, and quiet.

OTHER TIPS

- Cut back on coffee, tea, alcohol, and cigarettes.
- Take a warm bath or shower before bedtime.
- Exercise in the late afternoon or early evening, allowing at least a couple of hours between exercise and sleep.

Remedies

AROMATHERAPY

Lavender The aroma of lavender in the bedroom can help you fall asleep. Try a lavender sachet or a lavender pillow in your bed.

BACH FLOWER REMEDIES

White Chestnut: if unwanted thoughts keep you awake, try this flower remedy.

HERBAL REMEDIES

Chamomile Chamomile tea has long been used for its relaxing properties. Have a cup of chamomile tea before bedtime. Or try an herbal tea that has a combination of hops, chamomile, and passionflower. If you are allergic to chrysanthemums, daises, ragweed, or yarrow, we don't recommend using chamomile, as it may cause a similar allergic reaction.

Hops Usually thought of as an ingredient for making beer, hops has also been used for many years in Europe as a treatment for insomnia and nervousness. When you are having trouble sleeping, try taking two capsules of a freeze-dried extract of hops before you go to sleep. Hops is also available in tea form. Drink a cup of hops tea before bedtime.

Passionflower Passionflower tea can help you get to sleep. Although the exact mechanism of its action is unclear, the German Commission E has found it to be helpful for insomnia. Try a soothing cup of passionflower tea before bedtime.

Valerian This herbal sedative has been shown to be an effective remedy for insomnia. You can take valerian as a tea, a tincture (liquid) extract, or in capsules of the freeze-dried extract. It is usually recommended in the tincture (liquid) form. A few people are sensitive to valerian and may find that the recommended dose leaves them with a feeling like a hangover. If this is the case, cut back the dose or try a different remedy altogether. As valerian works like any other sedative, it is very important that you don't combine it with other sleeping pills, antianxiety medications, or alcohol. Be patient; valerian may take two to four weeks to become effective.

HOMEOPATHY

Calm Forts This is a classic combination homeopathic remedy that helps induce sleep. Try taking one to two pills one-half hour before going to sleep.

OTHER SUPPLEMENTS

5-HTP In studies, 5-HTP, a precursor of serotonin, has been shown to increase sleep at a dose of 600 milligrams per day. This compound is not recommended in combination with prescription antidepressants.

Melatonin A hormone produced by the pineal gland, melatonin helps regulate our sleep cycle. When it gets dark, the body starts to produce melatonin; when it gets light, melatonin production is shut off. This is why it is important to keep your bedroom dark so as not to disturb your body's production of melatonin. While some alternative health practitioners recommend taking supplemental melatonin, we don't advise this as a long-term solution for sleep problems. It can be helpful in the short term, however, if it helps you to develop a more regular sleep pattern. To help you sleep, the recommended dose of melatonin is 1–3 milligrams, taken approximately twenty minutes before your bedtime.

For some people, relaxation tapes are a way to turn off the internal dialog that keeps them awake. Try listening to soothing music or specially designed relaxation tapes to help yourself drift off.

Many community hospitals and health centers are developing sleep clinics to address the sleep problems many people experience. Be sure to look into local resources available in your area.

For Further Information

For more information on sleep disorders, contact:

American Academy of Sleep
6301 Bandel Road NW, Suite 101
Rochester, MN 55901
www.asda.org
(507) 287-6006

For more information on the complementary remedies discussed in this section, see chapter 3.

SWALLOWING CHANGES

Swallowing may appear to be a strange topic, but if you are having problems with swallowing, you will understand why it is so important to your well-being.

Problems with swallowing are often missed initially because the symptoms, such as weight loss or poor appetite, are attributed to some other cause.

COMMON SYMPTOMS OF PROBLEMS WITH SWALLOWING

- Steady weight loss because you are able to eat fewer and fewer calories
- Coughing when drinking and/or eating or having difficulty clearing your throat
- Experiencing pain while trying to eat or drink
- Suffering from another side effect or symptom of your treatment that is interfering with your swallowing

There are many reasons for having problems swallowing. Sometimes it is simply that you don't have the energy or desire to eat enough. Or there may be mechanical changes in your swallowing apparatus (saliva, tongue, gag reflex, throat, or esophagus) that make the act of swallowing a different process from what you were familiar with so that you have to relearn how to swallow. You may need to refer to another section in this book for ways to manage other side effects that may have an impact on your swallowing (see *Appetite Problems*, p. 57, *Cough*, p. 94, *Dry Mouth*, p. 118, *Mouth Sores*, p. 159, *Nasal Congestion*, p. 168, and *Nutrition*, p. 244). If swallowing is painful and you feel as though you have a constant sore throat from either chemotherapy or radiation to the head and neck region, upper esophagus, or center chest, see your clinician. If it is not infection but mucositis that is causing your swallowing problem, see *Mouth Sores*, p. 159.

Disease and Treatment Considerations

SURGERY

If your swallowing problem has to do with mechanical changes brought on by surgery to the esophagus, throat, or mouth or radiation to the mouth or neck area, you will probably benefit from a referral to a speech pathologist. Speech pathology is the specialty that deals with the mechanics of speaking and swallowing. Try to see the speech pathologist before your surgery or radiation treatments begin; this way, he or she can establish a baseline of your functional swallowing ability and thus will be better able to measure the changes that have taken place after surgery or radiation treatment. These changes in your swallowing function can be temporary or permanent. Putting in time and effort can make the difference in how you recover your swallowing skills.

CHEMOTHERAPY AND RADIATION

Chemotherapy and radiation can trigger some degree of fatigue, and feeling fatigued can certainly make eating and swallowing difficult. If you are feeling fatigued, eat your calorie-heavy meal in the morning. Then eat frequent, small amounts of nutritious snacks and/or meals throughout the day. We also encourage you to make sure that the fluids you drink include calories. This way, you get calories, nutrients, and fluids all in one package. See *Fatigue*, p. 122, and *Appetite Problems*, p. 57.

Mucositis   Certain chemotherapies, such as 5-fluorouracil (5-FU) and doxorubicin (Adriamycin), as well as radiation to the head and neck, can cause mucositis (an inflammation of the lining of the mouth and throat). Mucositis makes swallowing painful and difficult. See also *Mouth Sores,* p. 159, and *Dry Mouth,* p. 118.

Prevention

COUGHING WHILE DRINKING

If you notice that you cough or sputter whenever you drink fluids, we recommend that you tell this to your clinician; but you can also try thickening your drinks yourself. Thickened drinks are easier to drink. You can make thickeners by whizzing cooked rice in a blender to a liquid consistency and adding the mixture to whatever you like to drink. Or you can buy a commercial drink thickener over the counter at a pharmacy. Experiment with adding thickener until you find the consistency that is easiest to drink. See *Cough,* p. 94.

Remedies

FEEDING TUBE

When your clinicians expect that your swallowing, eating, and drinking ability will be severely hampered during treatment, they may advise that you have a feeding tube put in before your treatment in order to prevent you from having serious nutritional problems, dehydration, and severe weight loss. Feeding tubes are tubes used to bypass your mouth and esophagus. This tube will allow you to get the food and fluids you need even though you are unable to eat well. The tube goes directly to either the stomach or the top of the small intestine (jejunum) and can be slid down your nose or mouth for a temporary fix into the stomach or put in through your abdominal wall in a quick surgical procedure done under sedation. A surgically implanted tube is recommended if you need the tube for longer than a few weeks. We are told that feeding tube placement does not hurt and that a feeding tube can be used as long as you take care of it. You can live your life fairly normally, and you can even shower with a feeding tube in place in the abdomen. For more information on the options available to you with feeding tubes, discuss this with your clinician.

THICKENERS

If your swallowing problems increase, drink thicker drinks instead of clear liquids—for example, shakes, smoothies, or frappes. We also recommend that you sit up when you drink. Food and fluids must travel downward, and the easier you make it for them to travel down, the easier it is to swallow correctly. If your clinician is concerned with your gag reflex, a very simple test can be performed to check this. A visiting nurse can even do this test at your home. It's the "open your mouth and say ah" test where someone presses a tongue depressor on the back of your tongue and you gag. See *Dehydration,* p. 99, for more tips on consuming fluids.

SLOW DOWN

Another trick to eating, drinking, and swallowing is to eat with someone else. Company often encourages you to eat more slowly to be able to carry on a conversation and to chew in smaller bites. And, of course, socializing is very important to your well-being.

For more information on the complementary remedies discussed in this section, see chapter 3.

SWELLING

You can have swelling for a variety of reasons, not all of them related to cancer or to cancer treatment.

A common misconception is that swelling is caused by drinking too much fluid. Frequently drinking enough fluid helps your vascular system and kidneys to work better. Not drinking enough can worsen the swelling, because lack of fluids tells your body to retain fluid.

If you experience sudden facial swelling (especially around the lips and mouth) and changes in breathing, go to the nearest emergency room immediately.

Swelling is sometimes an inflammatory response. When your body suffers an injury of any kind, it sends many types of cells to check out and repair the area. This is not in itself a bad thing, but it can be painful and inconvenient, especially when the injury involves a joint. If you have swelling that is accompanied by redness, pain, heat, or fever, you may have an infection. In this case, call your clinician.

Diagnosis and Treatment Considerations

SURGERY

Lymphedema   Unfortunately, whenever lymph channels have been disrupted by surgery, including axillary (armpit) dissection for breast cancer, lymph node sampling for cervical cancer, and other abdominal or pelvic surgeries, there is a risk of developing swelling. This swelling occurs from lymph accumulating where the flow and circulation has been hampered by scar tissue. This side effect can happen years after your surgery and can range from merely annoying to debilitating. Lymphedema is a complicated problem that generally requires professional intervention and recommendations. We recommend that you discuss this problem with your clinician.

If you have had lymph node sampling in the armpit (axillary node dissection), it is recommended that this arm should never be used for blood draws, blood pressure, chemotherapy, or venipunctures of any kind. You should also try not to use this arm to lift heavy objects or to do heavy work. Protect this arm from cuts and scrapes, and don't play with a pet with this arm or hand. If you notice new discomfort in this arm, especially when accompanied with redness, warmth, tenderness, and/or a fever, call your clinician. Even if it is years since the procedure, call your primary care clinician and report that this is the arm on the side of your axillary dissection.

CHEMOTHERAPY

Swollen lower limbs, like feet, ankles, knees, and legs (edema), are a frequent problem after having medium- to high-dose cisplatin (Platinol) or cyclophosphamide (Cytoxan) for testicular, ovarian, or lung cancer. This swelling is caused by temporary fluid retention and is usually managed with prescription diuretics such as furosemide (Lasix). It is also recommended that you walk as much as possible and elevate your feet when sitting. Furosemide also signals the kidneys to excrete potassium. Discuss this side effect with your clinician. To increase the potassium in your diet, eat more apricots, avocados, beans, brown rice, fish, and bananas.

If you have new swelling in your face and/or upper body (especially with shortness of breath, a cough, and a history of small cell lung cancer), we recommend that you call your clinician immediately.

ADRENOCORTICOIDS

Swelling of the face is a common side effect of adrenocorticoids (cortisone, hydrocortisone, dexamethasone, methyl prednisone, methyl prednisolone, prednisone, prednisilone) and the chemotherapy docetaxel (Taxotere). This swelling is usually temporary and will resolve a few days after you have gone off the medication. Please be aware that adrenocorticoids should never be stopped without direction from your clinician.

ABDOMINAL SWELLING

Abdominal swelling (ascites) can occur if you have a history of colon cancer, ovarian cancer, uterine cancer, cervical cancer, abdominal mesothelioma, non-Hodgkin's lymphoma, or hepatocellular liver cancer. In fact, ovarian cancer is most often first detected because of abdominal swelling. Severe abdominal swelling is often accompanied by unrelenting hiccups (see *Hiccups*, p. 143), and increasing difficulty in breathing and eating. Temporary relief is often found from a procedure called a paracentesis, which can remove fluid that has accumulated in the abdomen. A paracentesis can be performed to help you breathe and feel better. Removing the fluid is usually not a cure for this kind of swelling, but it can sometimes provide temporary relief.

NIFEDIPINE (PROCARDIA)

Some blood pressure medications cause swelling because they lower your blood pressure by altering the way your heart pumps or because of changes in your blood chemistry. Calcium channel blockers such as nifedipine have this common side effect, often causing ankle and lower leg swelling.

Prevention

PUT YOUR FEET UP

Swollen lower limbs (where both limbs are equally swollen) not related to surgery are incredibly common and are most frequently related to inactivity. Very simply, veins transport blood to the heart. When mov-

ing blood from the feet and legs up to the heart, the veins have to counteract the force of gravity and depend on the muscles they are embedded
in to help them pump the blood back up
to the heart. This is why walking every
day can be helpful to your veins. As we
age, the veins lose their elasticity and
work less efficiently. When you walk, you
help your leg muscles to squeeze the
veins and push the blood up. When you sit, the blood pools in the lowest place on your body, which allows fluid to leak out and causes swelling
in the dependent part. This is why pregnant women are advised to put
their feet up as often as possible.

> *If you have new swelling in only one foot or leg, call your clinician immediately.*

To get gravity to help your feet and
legs, it is very helpful to get your feet
above your knees and your knees above
your hips to create a downward slope
toward your heart. Some people find it
convenient to do this at night while
sleeping. The best way to raise your lower
limbs in bed is to raise the bed itself. Try
putting phone books under the end
where your feet are so that your bed tilts
slightly down toward the head. Although
people like to pile up pillows under their feet to raise them up, pillows are
never enough; they tend to squish down, fall, or get kicked off your bed.

> *People often notice that their feet tend to swell up when flying in an airplane. If you are sitting for a long period of time with your feet hanging down, swollen feet are common, even if you don't have cancer.*

Remedies

HERBAL REMEDIES

Dandelion   The name "dandelion" means "lion's tooth," in reference to
   the sharp edges of the leaves. Dandelion has been used as a diuretic
   since the tenth century. Try drinking a cup of dandelion tea every
   day. If you can get fresh dandelion, you can eat dandelion leaves in
   a salad, although they are somewhat bitter; or try sautéing them in
   a little olive oil and garlic.

Nettle   This is another herb that is effective as a diuretic. Buy nettle tea
   bags, or steep three to four teaspoons of nettle leaves in a cup of
   boiling water. Nettle leaf is also available in capsule form (the rec-

ommended dose is 150–300 milligrams per day). We do not recommend attempting to pick nettle leaves yourself, as they can sting.

If you are drinking nettle or dandelion tea, be sure to include foods with extra potassium in your diet (apricots, avocados, beans, fish, brown rice, and bananas). Let your clinician know if you are using an herbal diuretic. Do not combine either with conventional diuretics.

NUTRITION

Poor nutrition and absorption difficulties can also cause changes in your body's protein levels. An imbalance of serum protein in the blood, known as albumin, can cause fluid shifts in and out of the circulatory system, allowing fluid to pool in your feet and legs. If you are eating poorly, you may not feel like doing a lot of walking, which compounds the problem of fluid shifts. If walking is a problem, try adding protein snacks and drinks throughout the day; but we also recommend you see a nutritionist for dietary counseling.

For Further Information

The National Lymphedema Foundation can provide you with more information about lymphedema. You can reach them at (800) 541-3259.

For more information on the complementary remedies discussed in this section, see chapter 3.

TASTE CHANGES

Certain medications and treatments can make food taste and smell different to you. Taste changes resulting from medication are generally temporary. However, sometimes radiation and surgery to the tongue can cause permanent taste and salivary changes. Keep in mind that people have different reactions to different chemotherapies and treatments, and what affects someone else may not affect you in quite the same way.

Diagnosis and Treatment Considerations

RADIATION AND SURGERY

Radiation and surgery to the nose, tongue, or mouth can change the architecture of that area and disturb nerves and cell function in your mouth. How this will affect your senses of taste and smell depends on where in your mouth the procedure is done. We recommend that you discuss the possibility of taste changes with your clinician before your surgery or radiation treatments begin.

Radiation   Radiation-induced taste changes can start as early as one week into treatment to the head and neck. These taste changes usually worsen as you continue with your treatments. Most of the time, some of your sense of taste will begin to return from three weeks to two months after head and neck radiation treatment is completed. This improvement can take as long as a year, and your sense of taste may not entirely return to the way it was before treatment.

CHEMOTHERAPY

These chemotherapies are reported to cause a metallic taste:

- Cisplatin (Platinol)
- Cyclophosphamide (Cytoxan)
- Doxorubicin (Adriamycin)
- 5-fluorouracil (5-FU)

Some people even taste the medication as the nurse injects it into the vein. These taste changes should start to return to normal about three to four weeks after the last treatment.

Remedies

VITAMINS AND MINERALS

Zinc   The role of adding supplemental zinc to improve taste problems has been studied in cancer patients receiving radiation to the head and neck. The dose being studied ranges from 18 milligrams four times a day to 45 milligrams three times a day while on treatment or after completion of treatment. We recommend that you discuss this strategy with your clinician.

Strategies We Recommend

- Rinse your mouth with saline solution (see *Mouth Sores,* p. 159, for recipe) or lemon water (a cup of water with the juice of half a lemon in it) before meals to neutralize the taste in the mouth.
- If possible, find foods that agree with the taste in your mouth.
- Most people find meat flavors to be the most difficult with taste changes. Hide the meat flavor in strong fruit-flavored marinades, or try basting meat in fruit juice before cooking.
- Be careful with foods with strong flavors. Try by tasting a small amount first before having a big bite.
- To avoid food aromas, try to get someone else to cook meals and food for you if possible.
- Eat food cold or at room temperature to reduce the impact of cooking smells.
- If you are having difficulties with little or no saliva or ropy saliva caused by radiation to the mouth, see *Dry Mouth,* p. 118.

URINATION PROBLEMS

Urination problems include urinary tract infections, burning and pain with urination, frequent urination, urgency (needing to rush to the bathroom), retention (difficulty emptying your bladder), and incontinence (inability to control your bladder). These problems can occur singly or together. Urination problems can be related to other health problems, as well as cancer.

FREQUENCY

Frequency is when you feel you are constantly needing to urinate, especially at night. When you get up more than once a night, or more than you used to get up, you are having a problem in this area. This could be the result of a UTI.

If your urinary frequency is not related to a UTI, we recommend that you avoid drinking large amounts of fluid three to four hours before you go to bed. We encourage you to drink two liters of fluid a day; however, we suggest you drink more of the fluid in the beginning of the day so that you won't need to get up to urinate when you are asleep. If you need to take a water pill (diuretic) in the late afternoon or evening, ask your clinician if you can modify the timing of it so that it does not take effect while you are trying to sleep. Be aware that the kidneys function at their highest efficiency when you are lying down, which is why you produce more urine at night.

If your problem is unrelated to how much fluid you drink, when you drink your liquid, or when you take your water pill, it can be related to stress incontinence or a retention problem (see below).

URGENCY

Urgency or urge incontinence is when you suddenly have a need to urinate and sometimes don't even make it to the bathroom in time. Like all of these urination problems, urgency can be a symptom of a UTI, retention, or even mild urinary incontinence. This problem can make carrying on your normal life very challenging, as you always need to be near a bathroom. People suffering from urgency often find themselves isolated in their homes and relying on adult diapers in order to go out. If you suffer from urgency, empty your bladder frequently on a regular schedule to prevent it from becoming overfull. We encourage you to discuss this problem with your clinician before it isolates you.

> *Whatever you do, don't stop drinking fluids. People with urinary problems often limit their fluids and risk dehydration. See* Dehydration, *p. 99.*

RETENTION

Urinary retention is when you are not able to completely empty your bladder when you urinate. This problem is often suspected when you realize that you have to urinate five minutes after you have just urinated. This is a frequent problem for men with enlarged prostate glands, men who sit to urinate, and menopausal women. The absolutely best way to empty your bladder is to do so standing up or squatting. We realize this is difficult for many people. This way the urethra extends directly down from the bladder and lets gravity help to empty your bladder. It is important not to rush the process of urination. Allow your bladder the time and relaxation needed for it to be emptied. Obviously, this type of urinary discomfort can be a problem for older men and women, whose bladder muscles may not be as effective as when they were younger. Mild retention often can be managed by urinating on a schedule, for example, every two hours, and by allowing sufficient time to relax.

INCONTINENCE

Urinary incontinence can occur as a result of many reasons (including childbirth, chronic coughing, excessive abdominal fat, and radical prostatectomy). Incontinence that occurs occasionally (when you laugh, exercise, or cough) is usually called stress incontinence. If your urinary incontinence is new, we recommend you discuss it with your clinician, especially if it is accompanied by new difficulties with walking or moving your bowels or incontinence of the bowels. If these problems predated your cancer diagnosis, there are a few different possibilities for repair, depending on the cause of your lack of control. Discuss this with your clinician. Mild urinary incontinence can often be managed simply by urinating on a schedule (for example, every two hours) and limiting your fluid intake four to five hours before you go to sleep for the night.

B_{12} DEFICIENCY

A deficiency in vitamin B_{12} (cyanocobalamin) has been associated with urinary incontinence. If you are a strict vegetarian or over the age of fifty, have your B_{12} level checked. If you have low levels of B_{12}, it is easy to correct the deficiency with an injection prescribed once a month. Vitamin B_{12} is found in meat and dairy products, but it is more difficult to absorb as you get older, because of other changes in the body. This vitamin is vital to the nervous system, which may be why it is involved in your urinary incontinence.

URINARY TRACT INFECTIONS

Men and women on cancer treatment tend to be more prone to UTIs. If you use a urinary catheter to help empty your bladder after surgery or are having trouble with completely emptying your bladder, you can also be more prone to UTIs. UTIs are also common among people who are under stress. UTIs are often unpleasant and can make you uncomfortable.

It can sometimes be difficult to differentiate between when you have a UTI or when you are having problems with urination because of your treatment. Sometimes your clinician may decide that treating the symptom as if it is a UTI is the prudent action to take and will prescribe an antibiotic. The diagnosis of a UTI can be confirmed by a simple set of urine tests that show whether you have too much bacteria in your urine.

Signs and Symptoms of UTIs   Pain with urination is also a common symptom of a UTI, and UTIs usually produce smelly, yellow urine. They can also cause a strong urge to urinate even if you have just emptied your bladder.

> *Menopause causes the acid environment of the vagina to become more base or alkaline, thus making the menopausal woman more susceptible to overgrowth of yeast and frequent UTIs.*

Disease and Treatment Considerations

BENIGN PROSTATE HYPERTROPHY (BPH)

For men over age fifty, changes in the prostate gland can interfere with urination. BPH is a normal condition of male aging. An enlarged prostate from prostate cancer can also affect urination in a similar fashion. Managing symptoms related to an enlarged prostate is best done with the assistance of your clinician.

SURGERY

Radical Prostatectomy   Urinary incontinence resulting from radical prostatectomy is a problem for which there are not many good remedies at this time. The "nerve-sparing" surgery has not been as successful at preventing this problem as was hoped. Kegel (also called pelvic floor) exercises, biofeedback, and surgical repairs are usually recommended for incontinence after prostate surgery. While you are working on this problem, we recommend that you consult the website www.diapersbedamned.com for good information on living with urinary incontinence. Men suffering with this problem are best advised to have a consultation with a urological expert in voiding dysfunction to learn about current research

> *The National Association for Continence publishes a series of fact sheets, including ones on prostate surgery and incontinence, that can be purchased for a small fee. Call (800) 252-3337 for more information.*

and what their options are for this problem. This is especially important for those considering surgical approaches.

RADIATION

With virtually any pelvic cancer (bladder, prostate, cervical, endometrial, rectal, or vaginal), painful urination can be a side effect of radiation treatment. Drink an eight-ounce glass of water mixed with 2 to 3 tablespoons of cranberry concentrate daily while you are on radiation treatment as a preventative measure.

Prevention

As always, we encourage you to take in as much fluid as you can so that your urine is virtually colorless and your bladder and urethra are well flushed.

CRANBERRY JUICE

A daily glass of at least three ounces of concentrated cranberry juice works well in preventing UTIs if you are prone to them. Cranberry is able to protect the lining of the urinary tract by interfering with the ability of the bacteria to adhere and cause irritation and infection. You can also take a concentrated extract of cranberry juice in capsule form, if you want to avoid the sugar often found in the juice.

STAY AWAY FROM SWEETS

If you have a UTI, try not to eat or drink too many concentrated sweets (candy, ice cream, sodas, fruit juice). A high sugar content in your diet can make you more prone to urinary tract infections by providing a food source for the bacteria, which feeds off the sugar. Diabetics are also more prone to UTIs for this reason.

PROTECTING YOUR BLADDER FROM RADIATION

If you are receiving radiation treatment to the pelvis, it is highly recommended that you try to keep your bladder full during your radiation treatment (if you are not on treatment for bladder cancer), so that as much of your bladder as possible is out of the pelvic radiation field. Before you arrive at the radiation treatment facility and while you get changed for your treatment, drink a large glass of water, and then don't go to the bathroom. Keeping the bladder full helps to push the bowel up out of the radiation field and can help prevent diarrhea from irritated bowel syndrome (see *Diarrhea*, p. 109).

> *A three-ounce or larger glass of cranberry concentrate can help relieve an irritated bladder during pelvic radiation.*

Remedies

BIOFEEDBACK

Biofeedback has been helpful for many people for learning how to control their incontinence problem. Biofeedback tends to be more successful with people who are detail oriented. Speak to your clinician for a referral for behavioral medicine if you are interested in pursuing this approach, as many insurance plans will cover biofeedback.

CONVENTIONAL MEDICATIONS

Phenazopyridine (Pyridium) Pyridium is a prescription medication used to relieve the pain and burning with UTIs. It is also helpful for relieving painful urination caused by radiation therapy to the pelvic area. Be aware that this medication can turn your urine an orange color and will stain clothing.

HERBAL REMEDIES

Nettle This herb is effective as a diuretic. Buy nettle tea bags, or steep three to four teaspoons of nettle leaves in a cup of boiling water. Nettle leaf is also available in capsule form. We do not recommend attempting to pick nettle leaves yourself, as they can sting.

Saw Palmetto In recent clinical trials, extracts from saw palmetto berries have been shown to reduce the symptoms of BPH. Compared with a placebo, men who received treatment with the saw palmetto berry compound experienced an increased flow of urine and a reduction in the number of times needed to urinate and found it easier to start urinating. The current thinking is that saw palmetto berries work by inhibiting the action of androgens and therefore exert an anti-inflammatory effect. A typical dose of saw palmetto is 320 milligrams of a standardized liquid extract, or two to three 600-milligram capsules, taken three times a day with food. Do not take saw palmetto if you are also using conventional treatment for BPH or while on treatment for prostate cancer.

Try the homeopathic remedy that best fits your symptoms. If it doesn't seem to be working after a day or so, discontinue it.

HOMEOPATHY

Abal serrate—for incontinence from an enlarged prostate

Cantharis—for when you have a constant desire to urinate

Causticum—for urinary incontinence that occurs when you sneeze, cough, or laugh

Equisetum—for any type of urinary incontinence

KEGEL EXERCISES

Kegel exercises involve squeezing the PC, or pubococcygeal muscle (the muscle you use to stop your stream of urine). Contract this muscle when you are *not* urinating, and try holding this contraction for a slow count of three. Relax for a count of five, then repeat. You should gradually work up to holding the contraction for a count of ten. To improve the strength of this muscle, try to do five sets of contractions three times per day. You can do this exercise anywhere, at any time. It is important not to contract the abdominal, thigh, or buttocks muscles at the same time you are squeezing the PC muscle. Both men and women can benefit from Kegel exercises. We suggest that you speak to your clinician about these exercises to ensure that you are doing them correctly. After doing the exercises, see if you can have your PC muscle strength evaluated. For women, weighted vaginal cones can also be used for Kegel-type exercises to help alleviate urinary stress incontinence. The cones are available in kits that include instructions for use.

For more information on vaginal cones, call:

Femina Kegel Cone Kit
Phillips Products and Services
(800) 705-5559

Kegel Weights
Self Care Catalog
(800) 345-7889

For Further Information
(For Both Men and Women)

National Association for Continence
PO Box 8310
Spartanburg, SC 29305
www.nafc.org
(800) 252-3337

For more information on the complementary remedies discussed in this section, see chapter 3.

WEIGHT LOSS AND GAIN

During your treatment, you will find that your weight is evaluated frequently when you visit your clinicians. Ideally, they would like you to maintain the weight you were at when you were first diagnosed or when you started treatment. Unexplained weight loss or gain is a serious problem for anyone who has a chronic illness and can indicate changes in muscle tissue or a nutritional imbalance. Your body needs energy and strength for healing that you usually get from your diet. Weight loss can signal muscle loss, because if your diet is not providing your body with the fuel it needs, your metabolic processes will turn to other energy storage in the body. Lack of physical activity can also affect your ability to heal, and muscle can deteriorate from lack of use if you are inactive. Weight gain can also affect your ability to perform daily activities and your sense of well-being.

Prevention

CONSULT A NUTRITIONIST

Cancer and cancer treatment can change your ability to eat and the way your body is able to absorb nutrients. You are well advised to see a nutritionist to get personalized information and strategies to cope with this problem. We can provide you with some general rules and strategies here regarding weight loss and gain; refer to *Appetite Problems*, p. 57, and *Nutrition*, p. 244, for more information.

Diagnosis and Treatment Considerations

WEIGHT LOSS

Most cancer treatments can cause weight loss. If you are not feeling well, it may be because you are not eating enough to maintain your weight (see *Appetite Problems*, p. 57, *Dry Mouth*, p. 118, *Exercise*, p. 223, *Fatigue*, p. 122, *Nutrition*, p. 244). You may also have another physical problem that causes weight loss (see *Aches and Pains*, p. 33, *Dry Mouth*, p. 118, *Heartburn*, p. 135, *Mouth Sores*, p. 159, *Swallowing Changes*, p. 197).

WEIGHT GAIN

If your weight increases, there are questions you should ask to pinpoint the possible source of the additional weight. Is this weight gain a sudden occurrence, almost overnight? Do you have a history of ovarian, colon, or prostate cancer? Are you noticing abdominal or leg swelling, new shortness of breath, or difficulty doing your regular activities? If so, call your clinician.

> *If losing or gaining weight is necessary while you are on active cancer treatment, we recommend that you do so under the supervision of a nutritionist who is experienced in cancer care, in collaboration with your treatment team.*

Did you just finish a course of chemotherapy? Did you recently have a type of chemotherapy that can cause fluid retention—docetaxel (Taxotere), cisplatin, cortisone, hydrocortisone, dexamethasone, methyl prednisone, methyl prednisolone, prednisone, prednisilone— or chemotherapy that requires substantial infusion of fluid, such as intravenous cyclophosphamide?

Breast Cancer For some reason, women and men on treatment for breast cancer often gain weight on treatment. This problem may be related to a general "blah" feeling people complain about while on their chemotherapy, a decrease in physical activity, or a constant queasiness that is only alleviated by nibbling on snacks.

Adrenocorticoids Fluid retention, and therefore weight gain, is an extremely common side effect of this class of medication (which

includes cortisone, hydrocortisone, dexamethasone, methyl prednisone, methyl prednisolone, prednisone, prednisilone).

Prevention

The goal during cancer treatment is to try to maintain your weight.

PREVENTION OF WEIGHT LOSS

Be sure to eat frequent small meals throughout the day. When you graze
more, you often eat more calories than if you sat down to three traditional meals. It is also a good idea for your snacks and drinks to include
meaningful calories and nutrients. See *Appetite Problems*, p. 57, and
Nutrition, p. 244, for more tips and suggestions to prevent weight loss.

PREVENTION OF WEIGHT GAIN

Try not to eat a lot of empty calories when trying to manage queasiness.
What we mean by empty calories are foods that are high in calories but
low in nutrients, such as doughnuts, French fries, crackers, and sodas.
All these calories start to add up. For example, gelatin is low in calories
but also low in nutrients. If you continue to gain weight no matter how
many sweets and other fattening foods you cut out, look at the fluid you
are drinking. Carbonated drinks are frequently a source of useless calories, as well as not being the best choice in fluids. We recommend that
you cut back on the soda and try to drink more water (see *Dehydration*,
p. 99).

- Don't get on the scale often. Try to weigh yourself only when you go
  to your clinician's office so that your weight is consistently meas-
  ured on the same scale.
- Wear loose, comfortable clothing. Dress in layers so you can put on
  items and take them off as needed.
- Try to walk every day.
- Snack on meaningful calorie items such as yogurt, cheese, nuts,
  whole grain breads, beans, and so on.

Remedies

EXERCISE

Add some type of exercise routine to your day. Exercise is any increase in physical activity. It doesn't have to mean going to a gym and pumping iron. Try to find someone to exercise with—perhaps there is someone in your support group? See *Exercise*, p. 223, for more suggestions.

MARIJUANA OR THC (MARINOL)

Many people have heard that marijuana is effective with nausea prevention and as an aid to increasing appetite. We do not recommend smoking marijuana, as there are definitely health risks to your lungs, esophagus, and mouth related to smoking anything. However, the active ingredient of marijuana, THC, is now available by prescription in the form of a pill, called Marinol. This medication has been found to be more effective when the dose is started low and slowly increased over a week or so to prevent what some people experience as an unpleasant sensation of euphoria. Speak to your clinician about whether THC is something that could help your appetite. THC is not recommended for the elderly, as it can cause decreased cognition. Some people do not tolerate the euphorialike side effect, no matter how it is dosed.

WE DO NOT RECOMMEND

Miracle Diets   We certainly do not recommend any so-called miracle diets that guarantee weight loss overnight. Most of these diets are designed for people who are not dealing with chronic disease. Novelty diets can be quite unhealthy in the long term and may prevent you from getting important nutrients you need for healing and well-being. Again, we recommend that you try to lose weight only under the supervision of a nutritionist experienced in cancer nutrition.

Herbal Weight-Loss Products   We also do not recommend any special herbal weight-loss products. Most of these products contain combinations of stimulating herbs such as ephedra, which can be dangerous for people with heart problems or other chronic conditions (see *Nasal Congestion*, p. 168).

For more information on the complementary remedies discussed in this section, see chapter 3.

Five

PRACTICAL ISSUES AND SOLUTIONS

IT IS EASY TO FOCUS ON THE PHYSICAL ISSUES THAT ARISE while coping with cancer; however, it is important to address emotional as well as practical issues. We have tried to highlight some of the more pressing issues that come up during this time and provide some practical solutions. Just as you are more than your body, the treatment you are receiving affects more than your body. Physical symptoms left untended can become serious problems; emotional and other issues can also become magnified if not addressed.

DEATH AND DYING

Most people have questions about dying and death yet are afraid to ask them. It is important to remember that death is a certainty for all of us, regardless of whether or not we have a cancer diagnosis. However, death can become a more immediate concern when you have a chronic and frequently unpredictable condition such as cancer. However, just because you have a diagnosis of cancer does not mean that you will die from cancer.

The first goal of cancer treatment is to prolong your life and keep it meaningful and productive. However, as much as everyone hopes to go into remission from cancer and stay in remission, this does not always happen. It is a good idea to think about your own death, even if this is not an immediate worry, as planning for this eventuality can help you to put your life in perspective and be sure that your time is meaningful to you. You should know that there are ways to make your dying peaceful and comfortable and the process of death easier.

Another issue to consider is what to do with your body after your death. Do you have feelings about cremation versus burial? Do you have ideas about your funeral or memorial? Do you have a will? Do you want certain people to have certain of your things? Or other people not to have certain things? It is advisable, although we recognize it is difficult, to take care of these issues when you are still feeling well. You can certainly do this privately, although we recommend that you write down your wishes accurately and sign and date the document in the presence of a witness. Let at least one person know where this document is in case it is needed.

> *The more information you leave behind regarding your wishes, the more comfort you provide for your loved ones at a difficult and emotional time.*

Important Issues about Prolonging Life

The decision as to under what conditions to prolong or not prolong life is perhaps the most personal and private decision you will ever make. There is no right or wrong decision; there is only the decision that is right for you. You can change your mind at any time, but please let those around you and your clinicians know your decision so that your wishes can be carried out in the way you see fit.

Should you have a life-threatening crisis, the decision whether to prolong your life should be made by you, not your clinician or your loved ones. If you want someone else to make this decision for you, you need to state your wishes concerning aggressive treatment clearly to your clinicians and your loved ones. Be sure to document your wishes in writing and in the presence of a witness to your signature and the date. Ideally, we recommend you get your signature on this document notarized. It is also a good idea to make copies of this document and to distribute it to and discuss it with those people you feel should have this information (your clinicians, your lawyer, your family, a close friend). This "living will" is not an official document in every state but can be very helpful for those around you to have if you are in a life-threatening situation.

The following website contains transcripts of an excellent show on end-of-life decision-making entitled *Before I Die: Medical Care and Personal Choices,* first shown on PBS in 1997.

Before I Die: Medical Care and Personal Choices
www.net.org/bid/
Thirteen/WNET, New York

Pain Control and Sedation

Not all people with cancer suffer from pain at the end of their lives, but for those who do, the biggest issue seems to be the misunderstanding that they will become addicted to painkillers. We want to reassure you that the need for pain control is not addiction. Cancer pain needs to be controlled and prevented by the appropriate use of opioid medications so that you are able to live your life as fully and completely as you can, pain free. Think of pain medication the way a diabetic thinks of insulin: that it is necessary for living (see *Cancer Pain,* p. 69).

End-of-life care often requires the use of medications such as opioids. A common side effect of opioids as the dose is increased is sedation. Elisabeth Kübler-Ross, a prolific writer on the process of death and dying, describes this increasing sedation as "practice" for those around the dying person to begin to let go. It can also be looked at as practice for the person dying to start letting go. This can be a very reassuring way to understand this process of frequent napping and drowsiness that can occur with the need for increasing the opioid dose. If you would like to be less sedated, it is also possible for your clinicians to adjust your pain medication to find a less sedating regimen with the same pain control.

Spirituality

Spirituality means different things to different people. For some people, it means belonging to an organized religious congregation, while for others it may involve personal spiritual practices such as meditation, yoga, or prayer. Whatever your religious beliefs are, when you are in a life crisis, it is important to let whatever you believe in provide you with comfort. If you have not been a believer before, you may wish to investigate spiritual practices now for the first time. As we write this, research studies investigating the power of prayer on healing are being conducted. The positive effects on health and well-being of having a spiritual life are also being researched. Reach out and talk to people about your hopes and fears. There are many wonderful books on the subjects of spirituality, faith, and what happens when we die: for example, *Peaceful Dying: The Step-by-Step Guide to Preserving Your Dignity, Your Choice and Your Inner Peace at the End of Life,* by Daniel Tobin (Perseus Books, 1999); *The Tibetan Book of the Dead* (Oxford University Press, 1974); and the classic *On Death and Dying,* by Elisabeth Kübler-Ross (Collier Books, 1993).

We believe it is as important to take care of your spiritual and emotional health as it is to take care of your physical health.

Dying

Dying is a process that you can have a certain amount of control over. Many people in the terminal stages of diseases die when they have decided to die. This means that people set goals that they are often able to meet successfully and then they allow themselves to die. These goals may never be shared verbally, but who has not known someone surviving against all odds to attend a wedding, a birthday, a holiday, or the achievement of a loved one? Many people with end-stage illness press their clinicians to give them an exact prediction of how long they have to live. The truth is no one knows exactly how long you have to live, but you probably have more control over it than you realize.

How Does Death Work?

Very simply, the human body has a very finely tuned and maintained chemical makeup. The different organ systems maintain this chemistry by supporting one another when necessary. This means that when one system is not working as well as it should, there is a backup system to pick up the slack. Then there are backup systems for the backup systems. These backup systems, however, can't do the job of maintaining the balance forever if the first system does not kick back in to do its job. When a person is dying, the various backup systems start giving out, and eventually there comes a point when this process cannot be reversed.

Our brains and mechanical functions control many of our body systems automatically. This is why it is possible to keep certain bodily systems working after the brain activity has ceased. For example, your lungs are under negative pressure, which forces an inhalation to occur to level out the pressure in the lungs. At the very end of life, the lungs will continue this function until all the other mechanisms stop. This is why it can appear to those around the dying person that he or she is struggling to breathe, which is a difficult and painful process to watch. The appropriate use of opioids at the end of life can prevent this mechanical struggle and gently prevent your body from struggling to breathe.

It is important to recognize that the dying person is still present until the moment death actually happens. We encourage visitors and loved ones to touch and speak lovingly to the dying person. It is recommended to share your feelings of love and grief and to reassure each other that you will each be all right. Does this help the person to die more peacefully? Who knows? But it certainly helps those who are grieving, and it cannot harm the person who is dying to let the person know he or she is loved and will be remembered.

Hospice

Hospice is end-of-life comfort care. The clinicians who work in hospice care are experts on caring for the whole person and their loved ones after the decision has been made to no longer pursue aggressive treatment. There are inpatient hospice units in many hospitals, extended care facilities, and nursing homes, and there are freestanding hospice facilities. Home hospice care, however, is the most common type of hospice care in the United States. Home hospice care is monitored and maintained by specialized visiting hospice nurses. A hospice nurse is the only authorized nurse who can administer intravenous opioids in a home setting, which can help a person to die comfortably at home. Most states also allow hospice nurses to "pronounce" death in the home. A nonhospice visiting nurse cannot do either of these tasks.

The other major difference between a visiting nurse and a hospice nurse is that a hospice nurse can usually visit as many times or as few times as needed by the person on hospice care. A hospice nurse will not live in the home, however, and cannot give twenty-four-hour care. If you or your caregivers feel you need around-the-clock assistance, you will most likely have to pay extra for this help or try to get a placement in an inpatient hospice facility.

When Is The Best Time to Change Care over to Hospice?

It is very helpful to think about the possible hospice care available to you, even if you don't have any immediate need for it. Discuss this option with your loved ones, caregivers, and clinicians. We recommend that the best time to engage hospice care is when you have decided that you have had enough in the way of cancer treatment aimed at cure. Most insurance plans, including Medicare, require that your clinician diagnose you as being within six months to one year of predicted death to be eligible for hospice. This time period can vary, depending on the state you are living in. Of course, there is absolutely no way to predict precisely how long you have to live. Don't worry. If you are in hospice care and you live longer than the limit, your hospice care is usually extended. We also recommend that you decide that it is time for hospice care when you are still fairly independent and don't need lots and lots of care. This way, you and the hospice care team (which can include nurses, home health aides, and social workers) have the time and leisure to get to know one another and to put together a good plan and a good team. If there is time to get acquainted, you and your caregivers will not feel as though there are strangers suddenly in your life when you need more care.

Home Hospice Care

If you are on Medicare or your insurance follows Medicare payment guidelines, hospice agencies, unlike traditional visiting nurse agencies, are usually paid per day, not by the number of visits. Therefore, hospice caregivers visit as often as is necessary, perhaps less frequently at first because you may not need them as much. As you become less independent, the hospice team often has the discretion to increase the care and visit you more often. Home hospice nurses are not private duty nurses, but they are available to help your caregivers keep you comfortable to the end. The hospice team is also available to comfort, support, and educate your loved ones and caregivers while you are alive, as well as up to a year after you die.

Getting hospice care requires that you have chosen not to be resuscitated if your heart or lungs fail to function. To be in hospice care you need to be finished with treatment aimed at curing your cancer, but sometimes you still can receive treatment to make you more comfortable, such as radiation or other therapies for pain and comfort management. We recommend that you discuss these issues frankly with your clinician and hospice team.

Finding a Hospice

To find a hospice near you, try the National Hospice Organization helpline at (800) 658-8898, or visit their website at www.nho.org. Another hospice organization, Hospice Foundation of America, can be reached at www.hospicefoundation.org or (800) 854-3402.

EXERCISE

Exercise is important to everyone's general well-being. While we don't mean you should run out and start training for a triathlon, we do suggest that you start to incorporate moderate physical activity, or at least movement, into your daily routine. This could mean doing a yoga stretch, taking a daily walk, or turning up the music and dancing. If standing and walking are difficult, adding exercise to your routine can be as simple as raising your arms or legs or doing a yoga stretch.

If you are someone who appreciates structure and can afford a financial commitment, a health club may be your best

Exercise has wonderful benefits. Exercise helps prevent depression and elevates mood, helps your bowels work better, can decrease feelings of nausea, and can even help you better tolerate cancer treatment.

choice for adding exercise to your life. If you prefer to do things according to your own schedule, however, you may get more satisfaction out of setting up and following your own exercise plan. Or you may benefit from hiring a personal trainer to get one-on-one instruction. It doesn't matter what you choose to do; just try to do something physical every day.

Adding Exercise

Find an activity that you like to do and that you will be able to do on a regular basis. By *regularly* we mean every day, or at least every other day. Whatever you choose to do, be sure to dress appropriately. For example, if you choose outside activities in a cold climate, wear layered clothing so that you can take pieces off and put them back on as your body temperature changes. If you choose to swim, be sure to have a robe or jacket at poolside to put on after drying yourself off well. Don't let your lips turn blue or your body shiver.

> *It pays to shop around when looking for a gym or health club. Don't forget to check your local YM-YWCA or YM-YWHA for programs or classes. There are also many instructional videotapes available that you can buy or borrow from your local library. Many communities also have adult education programs that include a variety of exercise classes.*

Getting Started

If you have not been much of an exerciser before, start slow and increase your chosen activity as you feel stronger. Remember the goal here is to move and to allow that movement to help you feel better. A good way to gauge how hard you are exercising is if you can carry on a conversation while you exercise. If you can't talk, slow down. If you are taking a class or receiving instruction in a sport or activity, let the instructor know about your limitations before the class begins.

When Not To Exercise

If you have known bone metastases or bone involvement (whether or not they are painful), we recommend that you speak to your clinician before embarking on any exercise plan. Pathological fractures can be a risk, and there may be some forms of exercise recommended over others for your particular situation.

> *If you have no hair on your head, cover your head to protect your skin and maintain a consistent body temperature.*

Listen to your body. If you are feeling too tired to exercise, don't force yourself. Exercise is meant to help you feel better, not make you feel worse. If you are not on cancer treatment, you can push yourself a little harder, but exercise should never be painful. If you feel pain or fatigue, stop. Pain is your body's warning to slow down and take it easy.

Walking

Walking is one of the simplest forms of exercise around, and it can be a meditative experience as well. Walking outside is relaxing, and the sensation of air and light on your skin helps you feel part of the world. Walking also helps the veins in your feet and legs to pump blood back to your heart. Walking can even help to relieve swollen ankles a little.

Yoga

Yoga is a wonderful exercise program for people undergoing cancer treatment. Yoga is done at your own pace, without competition, and has many benefits. It can help you lower blood pressure, increase relaxation, improve breathing, and maintain good flexibility as well as overall health and well-being. Try taking a beginners' yoga class, or take out a yoga video from your local library or video store.

No matter what form of exercise you choose, an important benefit is that it helps to preserve your lean body mass, which is important for overall health and well-being.

FEAR

For most people, *cancer* is a frightening word to hear. Although cancer is not the leading cause of death in this country (heart disease is), it is probably the diagnosis people fear the most.

It is okay to be afraid. But try not to let your fear paralyze you and prevent you from living your life as best you can, as well as making good decisions about what treatment you will pursue. Once you confront and name your fears, even if only to yourself, you may be surprised that you will feel better. Another way to deal with fear is by getting information. Learning about your diagnosis and exploring all your treatment options can provide you with some control over what is happening and help you make informed decisions regarding your care. We also encourage you to talk to someone else who has gone through a similar experience who may be able to help you gain perspective on your fears.

Support Groups

We cannot emphasize enough the importance of getting support and sharing your feelings with others. It may be difficult to share all your feelings with your loved ones, because they are so close to your situation, and you may be concerned about letting them know you are afraid. It can be incredibly liberating to listen to the experiences of others and to share your feelings with other cancer survivors. You don't have to go through this alone.

Support groups can offer understanding and advice from other people who are having a similar experience. There are many different types of support groups. Call the American Cancer Society, at (800) ACS-2345, or your local hospital for more information on disease-specific and general support groups in your area. If you feel up to it, you can start your own group. You can see if there is an interest by contacting local pharmacies, health centers, local chapters of the American Cancer Society, your local library or hospice, or by talking to visiting nurses. We recommend you consider including a facilitator who is not a member of the group but helps to focus discussion and maintain ground rules. For information on how to set up your own support group, a good resource is the American Self-Help Clearinghouse, which you can reach at (201) 625-7101 for advice and publications.

Yoga

Yoga is a wonderful tool to help you deal with fear. Because yoga teaches you to be focused on the breath and the body, the exercises take you away from your mind and help you to focus on what's happening in the present instead of worrying about what might happen in the future. Try taking a yoga class, or get a yoga tape from your local library or video store and try it at home.

Relaxation and Meditation

Almost any relaxation or meditation technique will also help you deal with fear. See *Relaxation,* p. 252, and *Meditation,* p. 242, for more ideas.

Bach Flower Remedies

Rockrose—for moments of fear or when you are troubled by nightmares
Mimulus—for specific fears, such as a fear of death or fear of the dark
Aspen—for vague fears of unknown origin

For Further Information

We recommend that you be sensitive to your feelings while gathering information. If something you read or learn is upsetting, stop and read something else. A good resource is the National Cancer Institute's Cancer Information Service at (800) 4-CANCER. The people who answer your call can talk with you about chemotherapy or any other cancer questions you have.

The National Coalition of Cancer Survivors is also a very good group to contact regarding information and support on being a cancer survivor. Contact them at:

National Coalition for Cancer Survivorship
426 C Street, NE
Washington, D.C. 20002
(202) 544-1880
www.nccs.org

The local chapter of the American Cancer Society may also be a good source for information and support. You can search for your local chapter at their website, www.cancer.org.

For more information on the complementary remedies discussed in this section, see chapter 3.

GRIEF

Grief is a common response to loss. There are many kinds of loss: loss of a loved one, loss of a breast, loss of your hair. You can also feel grief about the loss of your physical independence or the loss of the life you had before your cancer diagnosis. Cancer involves loss. It also brings you up close and personal with the knowledge of your mortality.

It is natural to grieve for the losses caused by cancer. In fact, studies on posttraumatic stress disorder (PTSD) have shown that suppressing emotions can have long-term detrimental effects. A famous study of the survivors of the 1942 Coconut Grove Nightclub fire in Boston discovered that the suppression of grief had profound effects on health and well-being and in some cases caused what we now call PTSD. It is vital to your well-being that you understand the positive power that acknowledging your grief can have on your wellness and ability to heal.

Grieving takes emotional and physical energy, but it takes more energy to suppress grief. When you are faced with loss, it is important to take the time to allow yourself to grieve for that loss. Your current feelings of grief may awaken old feelings about other losses you have experienced in the past. Expressing your grief will help you move on with your life (see *Anger,* p. 45, *Depression,* p. 102, *and Fear,* p. 225).

- Allow yourself to have feelings of grief.
- Share your feelings with others. It can be very comforting to find that you are not all alone in these feelings. Talking to others prevents feelings of isolation.
- Get counseling to help you cope with your loss, or join a cancer support group. Losses are common problems that everyone will face at one time or another.
- If you are having trouble sleeping, see *Depression,* p. 102, and *Sleep Problems,* p. 192.
- Don't let your grief stand in the way of taking care of yourself.

Bach Flower Remedies

Star of Bethlehem—is indicated for grief, emotional trauma, and loss.

Homeopathy

Ignatia—for sudden grief and anxiety

Staphysagria—for grief, especially in people who have emotions that they have long suppressed

Natrum Mur—for people who are easily hurt but don't like to express it

For Further Information

For people going through the grieving process, a good source of support and information is www.griefnet.com, which has links to e-mail support groups, a newsletter, and a resource directory.

For more information on the complementary remedies discussed in this section, see chapter 3.

HEALTHCARE DOCUMENTS

Paperwork is a necessary evil when you are undergoing medical treatments. *Informed consent, medical proxy,* and *living will* (also called *advance directive*) are documents you will be hearing about frequently. The more you educate yourself about these issues and documents, the better you will be able to understand the function of the documents and make informed decisions about how these issues and documents apply to your situation.

Informed Consent for Procedure

Understanding the concept of informed consent for procedure is a very important part of your healthcare. For example, on your way to the operating room or before you receive a blood transfusion, you will be asked to sign a consent for procedure. This form states that you understand that there are risks to the procedure that you are about to have done and that the risks have been explained to your satisfaction. Generally, this form is signed, presented, and discussed with you by the clinician who is to be performing the procedure. In the event of surgery, both the surgeon and the anesthesiologist should review their specific procedures with you and give you separate consent forms to sign based on the specific risks of each procedure.

It is important to read these consent forms through before signing them because they are legal documents and are part of your permanent medical record. However, these forms can be difficult for you to read precisely because of the emotional content regarding the risks involved in the procedures. An informed consent for procedure admits that the procedure may not have a positive end and may not work for you. The form may even list death as a possible outcome.

We recommend that you do not sign a consent form if you are disturbed by what you have heard and read. Now is the time to ask your clinician questions about what you have discussed and what you have read. It is important to resolve issues you are concerned about before you have the procedure described by the consent.

The only time an informed consent for procedure is not required is when you are receiving emergency treatment in an emergency room. In an emergency room, your consent and agreement are assumed. This is a very important issue if you have decided not to be resuscitated and you have arrived at the emergency room and are not breathing.

Medical Proxy

By federal law, all people who have been admitted to a hospital for any reason must be informed of their right to designate a medical proxy within twenty-four hours of the admission. Having a medical proxy has nothing to do with why you are at the hospital, although it can be a shock to have an admitting clerk, unit secretary, nurse, or physician ask you if you have designated a person who can act and speak on your behalf should you suddenly be unable to answer.

WHY DO I NEED A MEDICAL PROXY?

Choosing a medical proxy is not quite the same as making a living will, which is discussed below. The two documents have similarities, but they have different purposes. Be sure that you understand this difference, and try to keep them separate in your mind and in your papers. Completing a medical proxy form designates someone you trust to make the medical decisions *as you would have made them* in case you cannot answer for yourself. This person is supposed to make the choices that you would have made, not what he or she would do if in your position. This person is referred to as your medical proxy. Be sure to tell this person what *you* would want in a life-or-death situation.

WHOM DO YOU CHOOSE?

It is not recommended that you choose more than one person to be your medical proxy. It is best to choose one person whom you can trust to act as you would have wanted and to let others know that you have chosen this person and what you wish done, so that in a crisis, your decisions don't come as a surprise to others. You can choose a family member or a friend as a medical proxy. Sometimes people deliberately choose a nonfamily member, whom they believe will not feel as burdened by a difficult health decision. You can change this designated person whenever you wish. If you do not decide on a specific person as your medical proxy, the default person is usually a parent or a spouse. For example, even if you have been separated from a spouse for ten years and do not speak to each other, if you are technically still married, the law in your state may very well say that this person is authorized to make health decisions for you if you are unable to express them yourself.

Living Will or Advance Directive

A living will, also called an advance directive, is a document that testifies as to what you would want done in case of a life-or-death situation where you cannot communicate. Be aware that not all states recognize living wills and that you must have the correct document for the particular state. The medical proxy, however, is recognized anywhere in the United States. If you have a problem in a state that does not recognize a living will and you do not have a medical proxy who knows your wishes regarding resuscitation, the hospital, policeman, fireman, or emergency medical technician must do everything they know to keep you alive. If you have a medical proxy, that person can communicate what you want. If you have the proper documents, many states now allow you to prevent resuscitation measures from being made at your home even when someone has called 911.

"DO NOT RESUSCITATE" AND OTHER LIVING WILL ISSUES

A "Do Not Resuscitate" order (DNR) means that if your heart stops beating or you stop breathing, there will be no attempt made to revive you using cardiopulmonary resuscitation (CPR). It is possible to hedge a little on this issue by deciding that you want a DNR if what has happened to you appears irreversible but that you would want to be put on a breathing machine or have other "extraordinary measures" taken if your need for them is only temporary. Discuss these scenarios with your clinician until you feel comfortable with your decision.

A DNR order needs to be written by your physician into your orders *every time* you are admitted to the hospital. If you had a DNR written on the last admission, went home, and now return to be readmitted to the same hospital, even one hour later, you must have the DNR order rewritten.

Resuscitation is a complicated issue. Why your heart stopped beating or why you stopped breathing can make a big difference in whether a resuscitation attempt should be made. You will want to discuss this difficult topic very frankly with your clinician. Being resuscitated does not mean that you just bounce back to the person you were before. You can, but it takes time. Sometimes resuscitation means that you have been put on a machine or machines to keep you alive. The decision about resuscitation is incredibly important to make, and we urge you to do it before a crisis. We recommend that you have this conversation when you are feeling well and there seems to be no immediate chance of needing to act on it. Remember, nothing you decide on with your clinician is final until it is done. You can change your decision to be or not be resuscitated at any time. If you do not wish to be resuscitated, we highly recommend that you inform all of your clinicians and nurses and your medical proxy designate of this. (For more on resuscitation, see *Death and Dying,* p. 217.)

The last word on medical proxy and living wills is that everyone over the age of eighteen, regardless of his or her state of health, is well advised to think about these issues and designate at least a medical proxy. A crisis can happen at any time to anyone. Sometimes the best way to approach this issue with your loved ones is to have everyone fill out these forms together.

For Further Information

If you would like to get more information about these topics, the patient care representative at your local hospital can be a wonderful resource. Another resource for information about living wills and advance directives is the organization Choice in Dying, which can be reached at (202) 338-9790 or www.choices.org.

IMMUNITY

The immune system consists of special groups of cells, including T-cells, antibodies, and specialized white blood cells. The immune system also includes your bone marrow and your lymph system. Simply put, the immune system is what allows us to interact with the outside world. The immune system is like a surveillance system seeking out and protecting your "self" from what the immune system recognizes as "nonself." Your immune system is always working, monitoring your entire body for the presence of illness-causing bacteria and viruses. The immune system also monitors the body for cell mutations caused by diseases such as cancer, looking out for and removing cells that were once "self" but now are "nonself." This surveillance process may even have triggered the symptoms that led to your original diagnosis.

Diagnosis and Treatment Considerations

Surgery, chemotherapy, and radiation interfere with your immune system in different ways. All types of cancer treatment disrupt normal cell function and trigger the immune system's healing and repair mode. Chemotherapy can affect the bone marrow so that new blood cells are not ready to replace the blood cells being taken out of circulation. When large bones are involved in treatment, radiation can also affect the bone marrow (see *Anemia,* p. 40, *Bleeding and Bruising,* p. 61, and *Neutropenia,* p. 178, for a more in-depth discussion of this process).

Prevention

When you are on active treatment, you need to be very careful when using products that claim to boost immunity, because it is not truly possible to boost your immunity. What these products do is stimulate your immune system. Remember that infection, dehydration, and exercise can also stimulate your immune system. While you are healing or on active treatment, consider letting your immune system do its work on its own.

Probably the best way to let your immune system do its work is to limit your exposure to colds and flu by washing your hands well and using a saline nasal spray daily to wash viruses, bacteria, and dust out of your nose. Other excellent support for your hardworking immune system is to get enough calories, do some moderate exercise, and drink enough fluid every day (see *Appetite Problems,* p. 57, *Exercise,* p. 223, *Nutrition,* p. 244). And take good care of your mouth by gargling with salt water daily.

> *We recommend that you do not let children under the age of ten kiss you on the mouth or eyes or share their food. Ask friends and relatives with colds to visit you another time.*

GARLIC

Garlic is reputed in many, many cultures to be very helpful in the prevention of infection. Try to include more fresh garlic in your diet, or take odorless garlic as a supplement. When you cook with garlic, leave the peeled cloves out for fifteen minutes before you cook with them, as this enhances their effectiveness. If you find that garlic upsets your stomach, you can try taking it in a coated tablet. It is highly recommended that if you are having surgery, you cut back on your garlic consumption a few days before going in, as well as ginger, gingko, willow bark, and feverfew, as these herbs can lengthen the time it takes blood to clot. Do not take garlic as a supplement if you are on blood thinners: warfarin (Coumadin), aspirin, willow bark.

> *Good hand-washing: wet your hands thoroughly with lukewarm water, add a little soap, rub your hands together, especially between your fingers and the back of your hands, for a minimum of fifteen seconds, and then rinse off the soap thoroughly. Dry your hands on a clean towel. Bar soaps are easier to rinse off than liquid soaps.*

Remedies

HERBAL REMEDIES

Adaptogens   Adaptogens are "tonic" herbs. While some herbs have been found to be useful for specific complaints, tonic herbs are known for their ability to enhance one's overall well-being. Tonic herbs increase one's ability to resist infection and stress and increase one's endurance. Ginseng, ashwagandha, astragalus, and the Chinese mushrooms are all considered adaptogens.

ASHWAGANDHA   Ashwagandha (withanaia somnifera) is an Ayurvedic adaptogen. In one study in 1996, the results of which were published in the *Journal of Ethnopharmacology*, researchers in India found that in mice treated with cyclophosphamide, ashwagandha improved immune system functioning. Researchers believe that withaferin A, a compound found in ashwagandha, is responsible for this effect. The suggested dosage is 250 milligrams of standardized ashwagandha extract taken twice a day.

ASTRAGALUS   Used extensively in traditional Chinese medicine, the herb astragalus (huang ch'i) has been used in China as a complementary treatment for patients undergoing chemotherapy and radiation treatment. Astragalus has been reported to help the immune system deal with viral infection and enhance immune function. Astragalus can be taken in tea, tincture, or capsule form. A typical dosage is one to three 500-milligram pills taken three times a day.

CHINESE MUSHROOMS   Although it is not within the scope of this book to go into traditional Chinese medicine in any great detail, several mushrooms have been used successfully to help immune system functioning. We recommend that, if you are interested in taking these mushrooms, you see a traditional Chinese medicine specialist to get specific dosage and treatment specifications.

GINSENG   Ginseng is probably the most well-known adaptogen. Siberian ginseng was used by Russian cosmonauts to increase performance. Make sure to buy a reputable brand that has a standardized ginseng extract containing pure ginseng with no other ingredients, and take 100 milligrams twice a day. Do not increase the dose. Try taking ginseng for two weeks, then taking a week off. Ginseng is not recommended if you have diarrhea, poor sleep, high blood pressure, or diabetes. Ginseng is also not recommended if you are taking antihypertensive medications, antipsychotic drugs, digoxin, or any of the adrenocorticoids. There is some evidence that ginseng may have estrogenic effects and that therefore it may not be safe for women with a history of breast or endometrial cancer or for women on tamoxifen (Nolvadex). In addition, ginseng may interfere with the effectiveness of MAO inhibitors and St. John's wort.

Some lesser known adaptogens that can help support your immunity as you go through cancer treatment are listed below.

MAITAKE   The maitake mushroom (grifola frondosa) has long been used as an immune-strengthening tonic in traditional Chinese medicine. Maitake mushrooms can be eaten in food or as a supplement.

REISHI   This mushroom (ganoderma lucidum) is sold in capsules or in bulk form to be used in making tea. Reishi mushrooms have been shown to have antioxidant and immune-stimulating properties. Reishi may be taken in syrups, teas, tinctures, and tablets.

SHIITAKE   This mushroom (lentinan edodes), commonly used in Asian cuisine, not only is delicious but may help to support your immunity. It is thought that a compound in shitake mushrooms called lentinan is responsible for their supportive action. It is recommended that you do not take shiitake as a supplement or eat shiitake mushrooms every day if you are also on blood thinners, such as warfarin (Coumadin), aspirin, willow bark, feverfew, or garlic supplements.

OTHER HERBAL REMEDIES

Echinacea   Extensive research has been done on echinacea's immune-stimulating properties, although the research was not conducted on people who had a diagnosis of cancer. You can take echinacea as a tea, capsule, or extract (look for the standardized extract form). It is suggested that echinacea be taken only for six- to eight-week periods, as it may start to lose effectiveness after this time period. It is believed that echinacea stimulates the immune system you already have, possibly making it more sensitive to infection rather than increasing or building it. Think carefully before using echinacea while on active cancer treatment. Echinacea may be just too much for your immune system to handle, considering all the other work it is doing. It is recommended that you not use echinacea if you are taking adrenocorticoids (cortisone, hydrocortisone, dexamethasone, methyl prednisone, methyl prednisolone, prednisone, prednisilone), methotrexate, or any other hepatoxic medications or if you have an autoimmune disease such as lupus, rheumatoid arthritis, HIV/AIDS, or leukemia.

Milk Thistle Milk thistle (silybum marianum) has been shown to alter the cell membranes of liver cells by blocking certain toxins' binding sites. The recommended dose is 200–400 milligrams of silymarin (the active ingredient in milk thistle). At this time, there are no known side effects or contraindications for taking milk thistle while on other medications, although there have been reports of nausea, gastrointestinal upset, and mild laxative effects when people increase the dose of milk thistle too quickly. If you wish to take milk thistle, it is recommended that you start with a low dose and increase it slowly. It is not known if this herb is beneficial or harmful if you are on treatment for hepatocellular carcinoma (liver cancer) or liver metastases.

IMAGERY AND VISUALIZATION

Imagery is an excellent way to enhance your immunity. We all know about the power of images in influencing decisions and emotions through the effectiveness of advertising. Images, like dreams, are very personal, so it is important to choose images that are meaningful to you. For instance, you can imagine your cancer cells being swept away or erased. You can imagine a protective force, such as an animal or spirit, guarding your white blood cells or other parts of your body. You can imagine yourself, strong and healthy, doing an activity you enjoy. Or go on an "image vacation" where you can escape this reality for a period of time. Try using different images at different points during your cancer treatment. Specifying the image may work the same way that choosing the right remedy will work on a symptom. Experiment with images to find out which ones work for you.

MEDITATION, YOGA, AND RELAXATION

Any techniques that help you relax are going to help your immune system. Meditation can induce a physical state similar to deep sleep in which the body and immune system do repair work and healing. See the discussions of yoga and meditation in *Relaxation*, p. 252, and *Meditation*, p. 242.

VITAMINS

Antioxidants   Taking antioxidant vitamins (vitamins A, C, E, and selenium, among others) is often recommended as the first step to support your immunity. However, you should be aware that there is controversy among medical professionals about whether it is recommended to take supplemental antioxidants while you are on cancer treatment. While some studies have shown certain antioxidants could enhance the effectiveness of certain chemotherapies, some clinicians feel that taking antioxidants during treatment could be counterproductive, in that they may protect the cancer cells along with the noncancer cells. If you are taking antioxidant supplements, it is recommended that you discontinue them two days before until two days after each chemotherapy treatment to prevent any interference. It is also recommended that you discontinue antioxidant supplements during the entire course of radiation therapy, then resume them a few days after you have finished treatment. It is not recommended that you add supplemental vitamin E when on adrenocorticoids (cortisone, hydrocortisone, dexamethasone, methyl prednisone, methyl prednisolone, prednisone, prednisilone). We suggest discussing this issue frankly with your clinicians before you embark on your therapy.

> *It is well known that how you feel emotionally about your diagnosis and your treatment affects your immune system. Surround yourself with people you feel good about. If you are depressed, anxious or stressed,* See Anxiety, *p. 48,* Depression, *p. 102,* Meditation, *p. 242,* Relaxation, *p. 252,* Stress, *p. 264.*

WE DO NOT RECOMMEND

Fasting, Cleansing, or Detoxifying   Your body needs food for healing and repair when you are on cancer treatment. Now may not be the best time for "cleansing" or "detoxifying" programs. We recommend that you save these techniques for when you are finished with your treatment and have allowed your body to heal for a couple of months.

Epsom Salt Bath   When you are all done with cancer treatment, you may wish to try this gentle detoxifying bath. Add two to three cups of Epsom salts to a warm bath.

Vitamin A   Supplementation with vitamin A is not recommended for people with lung cancer.

For more information on the complementary remedies discussed in this section, see chapter 3.

MEDICATION SAFETY AND YOUR MEMORY

Memory changes can affect your personal safety at home and your safety when taking medications. If anyone around you has noticed significant changes in your memory, we recommend that you discuss these changes with your clinician. We also recommend some strategies to help you be safe.

Diagnosis and Treatment Considerations

Even the simplest treatment plan for cancer can involve complicated medication schedules.

BRAIN SURGERY

Depending on what area of the brain surgery was performed on, your ability to remember or perform instructions can be altered.

MENOPAUSE

The lowered levels of estrogen experienced in menopause have been linked to short-term memory deficits. Not much is understood regarding this symptom of menopause, but it is important to be aware of it.

SLEEP DEPRIVATION AND STRESS

Sleep deprivation, poor sleep, poor rest, and stress all definitely have an impact on your ability to remember and carry out instructions.

Prevention

Here are some tricks and aids we recommend to help you recall information and instructions you need for your health and well-being.

REMEMBERING INFORMATION AND INSTRUCTIONS

You have probably been advised to always go to clinician appointments with someone else. This is so that you don't have the burden of trying to remember everything that was said by yourself. This person can act as a second pair of ears. It is also possible to tape-record or make handwritten notes of your discussions with clinicians.

We also encourage you to write down the names of the different clinicians you speak with and what they do, to make it easier to remember who said what. Just recalling names can make a person dizzy.

SAFETY AT HOME

The Post-it note can come in handy here. Don't feel silly putting notes on the back of your front door reminding you to check the stove to see if the burner or oven was left on. Check bathrooms for sinks or tubs left running. Remember to check your pockets, handbag, or even your hand for keys to the door you are about to shut behind you.

PILL-TAKING AND OTHER MEDICATION RITUALS

Life certainly becomes complicated while on treatment that requires daily medication. Anyone who has to take a pill or medication every day forgets to do this sometimes. What can help you to remember? First of all, if you cannot recall whether you have forgotten to take a medication or not, it is recommended that you just forget about it. It is okay to miss a dose once in a while. If this is a medication that you take a few times a day, wait until your next dose and get back on track that way. It is easy to overdose without realizing it, and that can be quite dangerous. If taking your medications consistently is becoming a problem for you, we suggest you buy a pill box.

PILL BOXES

There are quite a few different types of pill boxes. We prefer the types that you set up once a week. If you take multiple doses of medication at different times of the day, see if it is possible to try to simplify your regimen. Do you really need all those medications? Do all your different clinicians know about all the various medications you are on, including your cancer treatment? When was the last time you saw each clinician who prescribed each medication for you? Once you have simplified your medication schedule, find a seven-day box that accommodates your needs.

The easiest method is for you or someone else to dispense your medications once a week into each slot. For instance, if you take the pink pill in the morning, put one pink one in each morning slot. For the white one you take three times a day, put the white one in each of the three slots of that day and so forth. This way you can see which ones you have taken and which ones you still need to take. Do not refill the boxes until they are entirely empty. This way you will prevent confusion as to what day or time it is and whether you have already taken that day's dosages.

WRITTEN SCHEDULES

For any complicated medication schedule, it is usually a good idea to write out a calendar with slots and the times of each medication you need to take with your treatment nurse. Put a little box next to the medication and check it off when you take it, or cross out the section. You can also write notes on the chart about how you felt the medication worked and if you experienced any side effects. Bring this paper back to the clinician's office to review how well the regimen worked.

We also recommend that you or someone else write up a medication schedule on a days-of-the-week grid. This can help you to know which medications should be taken apart from others, which ones need an empty stomach, and which ones go with food.

If you have another method for keeping track of things, such as writing a daily "to do" list, we encourage you to use it. It's important to use what works best for you to keep you healthy and safe.

Remedies

HERBAL REMEDIES

Ginkgo Biloba   Ginkgo has been shown to be helpful in studies with elderly people with known minor memory loss. One of the ways it is believed to work is by increasing the supply of blood and oxygen to the brain after you have been taking it for two to three weeks. However, it has not been specifically studied in patients with brain tumors or metastasis.

The commonly recommended dosage of ginkgo biloba is 40 milligrams of a standardized extract of 24 percent ginkgosides, the active ingredient, taken three times a day with meals. Regarding side effects, only occasional mild stomach upsets and headaches have been reported. Ginkgo seems to be more effective the longer it is used. It may take a few weeks to feel any noticeable effect. Ginkgo is not recommended for those on blood thinners or anticoagulants—aspirin, warfarin (Coumadin), heparin, feverfew, or garlic.

For more information on the complementary remedies discussed in this section, see chapter 3.

MEDITATION

When most people think about meditation, they picture someone twisted up like a pretzel into something called the lotus position. Let us begin by reassuring you that you can meditate in whatever position is comfortable for you and that allows effective breathing. You can lie down or sit up; you can meditate at your desk or on the bus; you can even meditate in the treatment chair while getting chemotherapy. We encourage you not to be intimidated by the idea of meditation. You don't have to be spiritual to meditate. You only have to be willing to try it and to keep doing it until you feel the effects.

Meditation may seem mysterious, but it is really quite simple. The idea is to focus your mind within yourself and be fully present in the moment. Most people already do this during certain activities without even realizing it. Whenever you are fully present in an activity, whether it is gardening, swimming, driving a familiar route, enjoying a sunset, or taking a bath, you are practicing mindfulness, which is a form of meditation.

Why Meditate?

Meditation has many wonderful benefits for your health. It can reduce stress, calm anxieties, and relieve fears. Meditation can support your immune system by inducing a physical state similar to Stage IV deep sleep. One of the most immediate benefits of effective meditation is that you are able to escape from the multitude of thoughts and worries that are constantly running through your head and experience what is called quiet mind.

Types of Meditation

There are many different types of meditation. Some forms of meditation involve a mantra, which is a word or phrase that you can repeat to yourself over and over to help you focus. This could be a word like *peace* or *love* or a word that has a special meaning only to you. It can also be a sound, like "Om." Other forms of meditation involve quieting the mind by focusing your attention completely on your breath.

There are many excellent books and tapes on meditation, or you can take a class. There are even Internet sites with visual images to help you meditate. Try one method, or try as many methods as you can find, until you find the technique that works for you. Remember, you don't have to do something esoteric to get the benefits of meditation; for example, prayer can be a form of meditation.

> *There is no right way to meditate. The right style of meditation is the one that you feel comfortable practicing and that you will do.*

A simple meditation technique using a visualization you can try right now:

Sit or lie down in a comfortable position.
Now,
    simply breathe.
Observe your breath.
Observe the air going in and out of your nose.
Be aware of your thoughts, but imagine them encased in balloons, slowly drifting up and away out of your sight.
Keep observing your breath,
    in and out.
Try to keep your breath slow and steady.
As more thoughts enter your awareness,
    (and they will)
let them float away in the distance, and
    let them go.

Meditation is a wonderful tool that can be used almost anywhere at any time

> *When you are ready to stop, stop. You can do this exercise for one minute or twenty minutes. Either way, your meditation will be beneficial.*

to bring you peace. You may start out only being able to meditate for a minute or two at a time. That is fine. Go at your own pace.

Further Resources

A good meditation resource on the Internet is www.meditationcenter. com. We find this site to be very peaceful and helpful with general information about meditation, as well as links to different rooms with instructions on how to try out the different forms of meditation.

GOOD BOOKS ON MEDITATION

Wherever You Go, There You Are: Mindfulness Meditation in Everyday Life, by Jon Kabat-Zinn (Hyperion, 1995); an excellent introduction
How to Meditate: A Guide to Self-Discovery, by Lawrence LeShan, (Bantam, 1984)

MEDITATION TAPES

Many meditation books are also available in audio format. Try listening to a cassette while you take a walk, or in the car, or as a daily practice. Another well-respected teacher of meditation is Thich Nhat Hanh. He has written several books on meditation, which have also been recorded and are sold in cassette format, including *The Miracle of Mindfulness: A Manual on Meditation* (Beacon Press, 1992).

For more information on the complementary remedies discussed in this section, see chapter 3.

NUTRITION

If you are interested in finding out more about nutrition, you can find many excellent books on nutrition and cancer at your local bookstore or library or through the Internet. We also strongly urge you to consider requesting the assistance of a nutritionist experienced in cancer nutrition to evaluate your diet and make suggestions and recommendations based on your particular needs and preferences.

Nutritional deficiencies can affect many areas of your life. See also *Anemia,* p. 40, *Appetite Problems,* p. 57, *Constipation,* p. 88, *Dehydration,*

p. 99, *Diarrhea,* p. 109, *Dry Mouth,* p. 118, *Infection,* p. 151, *Mouth Sores,* p. 159, *Swallowing Changes,* p. 197, *Taste Changes,* p. 204.

Nutrition is certainly a more complicated topic now that you have been diagnosed with cancer. Not only do many people on cancer treatment experience a loss of appetite, but determining what to prepare and eat can be a problem. Sometimes a cancer treatment changes the way you are able to absorb different nutrients, or because of possible treatment interference, you are advised not to take certain vitamins or minerals.

You may have to change your diet to tolerate treatment better. For example, a person getting radiation and the chemotherapy regimen 5-fluorouracil/leucovorin for colorectal cancer will be advised not to take folic acid supplements and to eat a low-fiber/low-residue diet while on treatment. Both of these suggestions are contrary to recommendations for the *prevention* of colorectal cancer.

Don't Believe Everything You Read

When you read articles and hear about nutrition and cancer in the media, you have to read carefully, as the latest nutritional information is most likely geared to the general public, not those with cancer. The remarkable discovery you read about may even be based solely on evidence from animal studies and, while promising, not yet proven safe for humans. For the most part, general dietary information is about the prevention of disease, not for people who are already living with a chronic disease such as cancer.

We provide general guidelines to the nutritional problems that can be expected with certain cancers and treatments. Don't forget to refer to the sections on specific symptoms for ways to manage and prevent problems with nutrition. If you need in-depth, personalized nutritional information or if you have other conditions, such as renal failure, diabetes, high cholesterol, coronary artery disease, gallstones, gastric ulcers, irritable bowel syndrome, ulcerative colitis, Crohn's disease, or any endocrine or metabolic disorder, we recommend that you see a registered dietician experienced in cancer dietary care and your other health problems.

A big problem with nutrition and cancer is that everyone you know is going to be giving you free nutritional advice and trying to get you to eat. The constant advice can get annoying no matter how good the in-

Try to eat a balanced diet. Don't eat foods that don't appeal to you, since eating is one of the pleasurable activities in life. Don't make eating a chore by forcing yourself to eat things just because they are "good" for you.

Fatigue is associated with cancer and virtually all cancer treatment. Try to accept help with meal preparation when it is offered. Cook simple meals to make life a little easier while you are on cancer treatment.

tentions are, and being forced to eat when you don't feel well can be very stressful. While what you eat is important, it is probably more important to keep eating. Keeping your calories up is vital to being able to heal and live your life.

We do recommend that you break out of the three-meals-a-day mold and eat more frequent small meals throughout the day. This keeps your gut working more consistently and often allows you to eat more than you would by sitting down to three big meals. No matter what you eat, drink water or other noncaffeinated, noncarbonated fluids to keep yourself well hydrated.

We generally recommend that you don't eat your favorite foods while on treatment so that you won't develop a negative association between particular foods and your treatment, regardless of what type of treatment you are getting.

Diagnosis and Treatment Considerations

Certain cancers, including colon, rectal, anal, gastric (stomach), esophageal, head and neck, pancreas, liver, and gall bladder, can make eating difficult because the cancer and the treatment directly affect your gastrointestinal system and absorption of nutrients.

LOW-RESIDUE/LOW-FIBER DIET

This diet is recommended for diarrhea prevention and control during lower abdominal and pelvic radiation. For more information, see *Diarrhea*, p. 109.

<u>MANY SYMPTOMS OF CANCER CAN AFFECT NUTRITIONAL STATUS</u>

For more information and specific remedies, turn to the specific symptom: *Aches and Pains*, p. 33, *Appetite Problems*, p. 57, *Bleeding and Bruising*, p. 61, *Confusion*, p. 87, *Constipation*, p. 88, *Dehydration*, p. 99, *Depression*, p. 102, *Diarrhea*, p. 109, *Dry Mouth*, p. 118, *Fatigue*, p. 122, *Fear*, p. 225, *Fever*, p. 126, *Grief*, p. 228, *Heartburn*, p. 135, *Hemorrhoids*, p. 139, *Infection*, p. 151, *Mouth Sores*, p. 159, *Nausea and Vomiting*, p. 170, *Numbness and Tingling*, p. 181, *Sleep Problems*, p. 192, *Stress*, p. 264, *Swallowing Changes*, p. 197, *Swelling*, p. 200, *Taste Changes*, p. 204, *Urination Problems*, p. 206, *Weight Loss and Gain*, p. 213.

Nutritional Problems While on Cancer Treatment

<u>CHEMOTHERAPY</u>

Chemotherapy is meant to work as a systemic therapy. It is administered intravenously or orally so that it travels throughout all body tissues to prevent or stop the spread of cancer cells outside the primary tumor location. Statistically, it is assumed that certain cancers and tumor cell types have a higher likelihood of spreading than other cancers, even if the tumor was completely removed surgically. We recommend thinking carefully about this concept before embarking on a nutritional regime meant to protect various body tissues, such as supplemental antioxidant therapy, during chemotherapy (see *Immunity*, p. 233).

Bleomycin, Daunorubicin, Doxorubicin (Adriamycin), Mitomycin, and Mitoxantrone These chemotherapies work by forming free radicals. Theoretically, then, taking supplemental antioxidants that protect you from free radicals may interfere with the effectiveness of these treatments. It is not yet known whether taking supplemental antioxidants (vitamins A, C, E, beta-carotene, flavonoids, selenium) interferes with the effectiveness of these chemotherapies. At the time of this writing, it is believed to be wise to refrain from taking supplemental antioxidants for at least two to three days before and after the chemotherapy infusion.

Cisplatin (Platinol) Especially in high doses, cisplatin depletes magnesium stores in your body. If you are on this chemotherapy, your clinician will monitor your blood levels of magnesium. Do not be surprised if you need to get a magnesium solution administered intravenously. If your serum magnesium levels are low while you are on treatment, intravenous magnesium is actually more effective in improving the level than just getting magnesium through food. You can also add supplemental magnesium to your diet (start with an additional 100 milligrams per day) or increase your intake of foods rich in magnesium such as nuts, nut butters, peas and beans, whole wheat bread and cereals, cornmeal, shredded wheat, oatmeal, Brewer's yeast, wheat germ, cocoa, bitter chocolate, instant coffee or tea, and blackstrap molasses. If you are on cisplatin, try to limit the amount of calcium-rich foods you eat. To absorb the magnesium from foods better, don't eat calcium-rich foods such as milk, yogurt, cheese, dark leafy vegetables, sardines, and broccoli at the same time as magnesium-rich foods.

Vitamin B_6 It is recommended that you do not take supplemental B_6 while on cisplatin, as it may interfere with the effectiveness of the cisplatin.

Adrenocorticoids These medications (cortisone, hydrocortisone, dexamethasone, methyl prednisone, methyl prednisolone, prednisone, prednisilone) all increase the secretion of hydrochloric acid in the stomach, irritating the protective lining in the esophagus and stomach. This can leave you with gastric reflux (heartburn) and stomach upset, especially if you take them on an empty stomach. See *Heartburn,* p. 135, for more remedies and information. On the other hand, steroids can also stimulate your appetite in the short term. We recommend that you choose your snacks carefully while on these medications and always take these medications with food.

The adrenocorticoids can also cause fluid retention while signaling the kidneys to excrete potassium and calcium out through your urine. We recommend that you increase these minerals only through food sources, for example, by eating yogurt. If you are on steroids, it is not recommended that you take supplemental calcium or potassium unless specifically directed to do so by your clinician.

Coenzyme Q10 Coenzyme Q10 may also interfere with the effectiveness of these chemotherapies because of its potent antioxidant capability. It may be advisable to stop taking coenzyme Q10 until you are done with treatment.

Leucovorin and Methotrexate   It is recommended that you do not take additional folate or folic acid while on these chemotherapies because the folic acid competes with them at the cellular level, preventing them from working. You may also choose to cut back on folate-rich foods such as beans, spinach, fortified oatmeal, wheat germ, broccoli, asparagus, Brussels sprouts, peas, corn, and avocados.

Procarbazine   Procarbazine *must never* be combined with alcohol. This is a very serious warning. While on procarbazine, you must also avoid food and drinks containing tyramine. Tyramine can be found in beer, wine, aged cheese, Brewer's yeast, chicken liver, and bananas. Combining any of these foods in any amount with procarbazine can cause life-threatening reactions. Be sure to read the labels on prepared foods very carefully, and if you have a question about a particular food, do not eat or drink the product *until at least two weeks after* you are completely done with procarbazine treatment. Since St. John's wort has been shown to be chemically similar to an MAO inhibitor, it is also recommended that you avoid St. John's wort while on procarbazine.

RADIATION

Radiation creates free radicals. As in the case of the chemotherapies that form free radicals (see above), it may not be a good idea to take supplemental antioxidants (vitamins A, C, and E, beta-carotene, coenzyme Q10, flavonoids, or selenium) to protect yourself from these free radicals for the duration of your radiation therapy course. As far as is known at the time of this writing, eating the foods that contain these nutrients in moderate amounts is probably safe during treatment.

OTHER MEDICATIONS COMMONLY USED DURING CANCER TREATMENT

Trimethoprim-sulfamethoxazol (Bactrim) is a common antibiotic used in cancer care, especially after bone marrow and stem cell transplants. It is also the standard antibiotic prescribed for urinary tract infections. Bactrim depletes folic acid in the body. If you are taking Bactrim, it is advised that you take supplemental folic acid or folate, if this is not contraindicated by other medications, such as leucovorin or methotrexate.

NUTRITIONAL SUPPLEMENTS

There seem to be more and more nutritional and dietary supplements, liquid and bar, available in pharmacies and supermarkets these days. The differences between them are the amount of protein per calorie, whether they include cow or soy milk, and how much sweetener (calories) they contain. Please be aware that the brand-name formulas and bars can be quite expensive. Whether you want to use these supplements or not is a matter of your own personal preference. The key here is to remember that these products are nutritional *supplements;* in other words, they are to be consumed *in addition to* your normal diet, not instead of food. You are much better off getting your nutrients from a varied diet. Nutritional supplements are excellent to use as snacks if the frequent small meals we recommend are difficult for you. If you cannot eat, and liquid supplements are the only thing you can get down, we recommend that you seek the help of your clinician or a cancer nutritionist to help make sure that you are getting enough calories and nutrients.

These types of nutritional drinks and bars are only recommended as an addition to your diet. You can try adding a supplement after your evening meal or as a snack between meals. This will add calories and nutrients and usually will not interfere with your appetite at your regular mealtime.

PROTEIN

To increase the protein content of food, as well as add calories, sprinkle powdered milk or soy protein powder on foods. Add butter, sour cream, yogurt, cheese, or tofu to your diet, as long as you are not trying to avoid calcium. Try making instant breakfast drinks with half as much milk or soy milk so that you get more nutrients in a smaller amount of fluid. These drinks tend to be very sweet, so be sure you like that sort of thing.

YOGURT SMOOTHIES

Yogurt smoothies are very easy to make in a blender. Just fill the blender with any fresh fruit and yogurt and blend. You can include wheat germ in this concoction to add additional roughage and vitamin B6. Yogurt is unlike other dairy products because of the live bacteria it contains and is usually well tolerated, even by those who have gastrointestinal problems with other dairy foods. Yogurt is also an excellent source of calcium and potassium. Try to buy whole milk yogurt for more calories and more effective live bacteria. Unless you are neutropenic, be sure to use the yogurt with live bacteria, since it's good for you.

WE DO NOT RECOMMEND

Macrobiotic Diet   We don't advocate a macrobiotic diet because it's a very energy-consuming diet to maintain, especially when you aren't feeling well. A macrobiotic diet is generally low in calories and fat content. This translates to having to eat large quantities of food to get enough calories. When you are finished with cancer treatment and are feeling more like yourself, go ahead and try this diet if you like. If you are interested in this diet, the Macrobiotic Society recommends participation in a weekend introductory course where you learn the concepts behind the diet, as well as cooking tips. For more information about the macrobiotic diet, you can visit www.macrobiotic.org.

High-Protein Drinks   We do not recommend the high-protein muscle-building drinks that you can purchase in health food and vitamin stores. They are loaded with megadoses of vitamins, minerals, and protein that your body probably does not need. Remember that your kidneys and liver are basically in charge of clearing medications out of your body, as well as the storage and clearance of vitamins, minerals, and protein. You might not want to overload those systems at this time.

Tobacco and Alcohol   It almost goes without saying that tobacco use and excessive alcohol consumption can interfere with your body's ability to absorb nutrients and to function efficiently. If you can't stop these activities while on treatment, try to cut back as much as you can.

Electrolyte Drinks   We also do not recommend electrolyte-rich drinks (Gatorade, Pedia-lyte, etc.) unless they have been recommended to you by your clinician. These drinks don't contain much in the way of actual nutrition or calories. It is easy to fill up on them and then not be able to eat enough food. We do advise that you keep drinking liquids, such as soups and fruit juices diluted with water.

For more information on the complementary remedies discussed in this section, see chapter 3.

RELAXATION

If you are like most people, being told to relax only makes you tense up more. We are not suggesting that relaxation is easy, but on the other hand, it's probably not as difficult as you imagine. Learning relaxation techniques can have an enormous positive impact on your mental and physical health.

Relaxation is like any other skill you may have learned or taught yourself—you need to give it some time and practice to work. Relaxation is not effortless. It involves a conscious attempt at getting your body to let go of tension. Please see *Meditation*, p. 242, as relaxation and meditation truly go hand in hand.

Diagnosis and Treatment Considerations

For many relaxation techniques, lying down flat on your back is considered one of the most supportive and relaxing positions, as it allows you to release the tension in your back, neck, and shoulders. However, some people may not be able to lie down flat or to lie down at all. If lying flat is a problem for you, try different positions until you find the position that suits the type of relaxation practice you have chosen. Once you have had some practice at relaxation exercises, you may find that you can use these tools to relax in any position or place.

SOURCES OF INFORMATION

Some people benefit from formal classes to learn relaxation techniques, while other people prefer to learn methods on their own. Use whatever relaxation technique works for you. Browse through our suggestions and try something that appeals to you. We are presenting only a few relaxation techniques; many more types are available.

RELAXATION TAPES

You can find relaxation tapes in bookstores, alternative health stores, or even museum and nature stores found in malls. Some of these tapes prompt you through a relaxation or meditation process, while others have repetitive sounds. Some tapes have music that is written in a specific number of beats per minute, which has been shown to subliminally help breathing. Relaxation tapes can be a good choice for the person who feels he or she cannot relax, no matter what. Try listening to a tape and bliss out.

MUSIC

Some people have a particular composer, performer, or recording that allows them to zone out. Don't be afraid to use what works. The idea is to allow yourself to relax. How you get there is immaterial.

YOGA

Yoga is one of the most popular and effective relaxation techniques. *Yoga* is the generic term for a number of different mind/body disciplines from India. We recommend hatha yoga for its emphasis on breathing and its gentle, noncompetitive approach. You can do yoga on your own or in a class. If you have physical limitations, we recommend that you seek a class where you can learn alternatives to the standard positions or learn other modifications that will be helpful to you. There are many good yoga books and videos on the market. For more information and to buy tapes and books directly, you can contact the American Yoga Association at (941) 927-4977. Another good place to buy yoga tapes, books, and accessories is the website of the magazine *Yoga Journal,* www.yogajournal.com. If you don't have access to a yoga class, you can take out a book on yoga at the public library. You don't have to be a human rubber band to do yoga and feel its benefits. Yoga is meant to be noncompetitive, even with yourself.

> *In a 1997 study of thirty-three cancer patients undergoing chemotherapy, patients reported that music helped them deal with their loneliness during treatment and kept their anxiety under control. Listening to the music of their choice also made the time spent undergoing chemotherapy go by faster.*

Savasana One healing yoga pose is called *Savasana,* also known as corpse pose (don't let the name put you off). In this pose, you lie on your back on a mat with your arms a few inches away from your body. Your palms are facing upward, your feet comfortably apart. You may want to put a blanket or a towel over yourself to stay warm. Exhale and let your body sink into the ground. You will probably feel tension somewhere in your body. Try to release this tension by breathing slowly into any tight spots you can find. Try to release any emotional tension, as well as any unwanted thoughts. Stay quietly in the pose for as long as you wish, breathing slowly and deeply.

EXERCISE

Regular exercise is also a wonderful relaxation tool. It increases your heart rate, provides you with a change of scenery, and can be a social experience. Walking and swimming are two terrific ways to clear your mind and relieve stress.

BIOFEEDBACK

If you have difficulty learning traditional relaxation methods, biofeedback may be for you. Biofeedback teaches you to monitor and learn how to change body functions such as heart rate, blood pressure, and muscle tension, using machines that let you know your progress. Generally, biofeedback training consists of ten weekly hour-long sessions. Medical insurance may cover some of the cost of biofeedback. We recommend that if you have a pacemaker, you check with your clinician before beginning biofeedback training.

PROGRESSIVE RELAXATION

One technique you can try on your own is *progressive relaxation*—a term coined by psychologist Edmund Jacobson and popularized by Herbert Benson. This technique is a great way to relax and reduce anxiety. Another plus is that it can be done while lying down or sitting up. Start by making yourself comfortable, but supported, in good body alignment. Cover yourself with a blanket or towel (as your body temperature may drop slightly). Then, slowly and methodically, go through each part of your body, one at a time, starting with the toes (the progression is toes, feet, legs, buttocks, stomach, rib cage, shoulders, arms, hands, face, forehead, scalp, jaw, mouth). Tense each part for a few seconds, and then tell yourself to release all the tension in that part of your body. Keep reminding yourself to breathe. After you have gone through your whole body, tensing and releasing each part, imagine a healing white light slowly traveling up and filling your body, from the tips of your toes to the top of your head. When the light reaches the top of your head, let the light push any negative thoughts and tension out the top of your head. Just let them go. Then close your eyes and enjoy the positive effects of this exercise for a few moments. Before you get up, wiggle and stretch your various body parts (as you see cats and babies do before they get up).

HYPNOSIS

Hypnosis is a special state of consciousness, a state of deep relaxation where you become more open to the power of suggestion. Don't worry, you won't do anything under hypnosis that you wouldn't do otherwise. Some examples of the benefits of hypnosis for people facing cancer can be the reduction of stress and pain. When hypnotized, you can give yourself the suggestion that you are going to feel healthy and strong after your chemo, or imagine yourself doing an activity you love in the future. Hypnosis works for some people and not for others. Don't do hypnosis if the idea makes you feel uncomfortable.

SPIRITUALITY

Some people feel peace and relief after participating in a religious ceremony or another kind of spiritual activity. Keep in mind that your spiritual wellness can be very important to your health.

NUTRITION

Cut back on stimulants (coffee, green and black tea, and caffeinated sodas) when you are trying to relax. Instead, drink hot water with lemon, or herbal teas known for their relaxing effects, such as chamomile or passionflower. We recommend no more than two cups a day of each type of herbal tea. If you are allergic to chrysanthemums, daises, ragweed, or yarrow, we don't recommend using chamomile, as it may cause a similar allergic reaction.

> *Try to eat more carbohydrates every day. Carbohydrates such as potatoes, bread, and pasta can have a calming effect.*

See *Anxiety*, p. 48, and *Stress*, p. 264, for more suggestions.

AROMATHERAPY

Three aromatherapy oils that help induce relaxation are lavender, geranium, and marjoram. You can keep a tiny vial of one of these essential oils with you and inhale as needed, or put a few drops into a vaporizer or the water of a relaxing warm bath. Geranium is not recommended while you are on active treatment as it may overstimulate the endocrine system.

WE DO NOT RECOMMEND

We do not recommend relying on alcohol or marijuana for relaxation purposes.

Further Resources

YOGA

To learn more about yoga and to learn simple yoga positions by viewing pictures, try www.yogaclass.com. You can click on a topic such as "relax" or "workout," and the site will guide you through a series of postures with suggestions on how to get the most out of them.

RELAXATION RESPONSE

To learn more about the relaxation response, read Herbert Benson's *Relaxation Response* or his more recent book, *Beyond the Relaxation Response: How to Harness the Healing Power of Your Personal Beliefs.*

HYPNOSIS

To find a professional hypnotist near you, call the American Council of Hypnotist Examiners, at (818) 242-5378, or the American Institute of Hypnotherapy, at (714) 261-6400.

BIOFEEDBACK

To find a certified biofeedback instructor, you can call the Biofeedback Certification Institute of America at (303) 420-2902 or search their database at www.bcia.org.

For more information on the complementary remedies discussed in this section, see chapter 3.

SEX AND SEXUALITY

Sexuality is an integral part of being human, and sex is one of the ways we express ourselves in intimate relationships. Sexual health is also a subject many people find difficult to discuss with anyone, including their clinicians. You may feel that, given the seriousness of your diagnosis and treatment, your sexual health should not be a concern, but we would like to encourage you to remember that your sexual health can have an impact on your overall well-being.

Intimacy

If you are having difficulty dealing with intimacy and your feelings about intimate relationships, we suggest that you refer to our sections on *Anger*, p. 45, *Anxiety*, p. 48, *Depression*, p. 102, *Fear*, p. 225, *Grief*, p. 228, *Meditation*, p. 242, *Relaxation*, p. 252, and *Stress*, p. 264. We also recommend working with a mental health counselor for support and reassurance regarding these issues.

> *Sex may be a very difficult issue for you to bring up with your partner or potential partners, but communication is the way to any healthy intimate relationship. We recommend that you do not assume anything about your partner's feelings. Let your partner express himself or herself.*

Was Sexuality a Difficult Issue before Cancer?

If you were having difficulties in your sex life before cancer, these problems may be intensified now. You may need to seek the help of a professional counselor, preferably one who is experienced in sex counseling and the issues surrounding a cancer diagnosis.

Normal Sex?

There is no such thing as normal sex. Sex is what feels right to you. Masturbating is sex. Touching and fondling are sexual acts. Give yourself time to adjust to the way your body feels after treatment. Sometimes you may need to reassure your partner that you still desire sex and intimacy.

> *Cancer cannot be caught through sexual contact.*

Desire and Libido

Give yourself and your partner some time to adjust to the changes cancer can bring. Don't be afraid to talk about your feelings and ask your clinicians questions. Remember that it may take time for your desire for sex to return. However, if your lack of interest in sex continues, it can be a sign of depression, which can be treated.

Emotions

Virtually any emotional problem can affect your sexual health. Once you have addressed an emotional issue, you may find that your feelings about sex improve. Please refer to *Anger,* p. 45, *Anxiety,* p. 48, *Depression,* p. 102, *Fear,* p. 225, *Grief,* p. 228, and *Stress,* p. 264.

Diagnosis and Treatment Considerations

One thing we would really like you to keep in mind is that being intimate sexually will not interfere with your cancer treatment's effectiveness. Unless your clinician advises you otherwise, it is generally safe to engage in sexual or intimate activity while you are under treatment.

SURGERY

Physical Changes   Physical changes can have a profound effect on your sexual health. We encourage you to address these issues directly to find a way to recover a sense of control over who you are and what you look like. There are organizations you can contact that can help you deal with these changes. Here are a few.

Look Good, Feel Better
c/o American Cancer Society
(800) ACS-2345
www.lookgoodfeelbetter.org

National Prostate Cancer Coalition
1300 19th Street, NW, Suite 400
Washington, D.C. 20036
(813) 253-0541
www.4npcc.org

United Ostomy Association
19772 MacArthur Boulevard, Suite 200
Irvine, CA 92612
(800) 826-0826
www.uoa.org

Y-Me Breast Cancer Organization
212 West Van Buren Street
Chicago, IL 60607
(800) 221-2141
www.y-me.org

CHEMOTHERAPY

The systemic cancer therapies, including chemotherapy, hormone therapy, and biological response modifiers, can all interfere with sexual response and cause temporary, although disturbing, physical changes that can affect sexual functioning and intimacy in both men and women. Side effects of treatment that directly affect sexual health run the gamut from physical pain and hair loss to weight gain. These changes can be even more of a problem because their impact on sexual health is so rarely directly addressed by patients or clinicians.

THROMBOCYTOPENIA AND NEUTROPENIA

When you have low platelets or low white blood cell counts, sexual intercourse is not recommended, because you will have a lower threshold for bruising and are at greater risk for infection until your counts come back up. See *Bleeding and Bruising,* p. 61, and *Neutropenia,* p. 178, for more information on these topics.

BIRTH CONTROL

We recommend that you and your partner use condoms while you are on any systemic cancer therapy not only on the day you receive the infusion but for forty-eight hours afterward. This method not only prevents pregnancy but also protects you and your partner from minute amounts of the treatment medication that may still be present in your bodily fluids.

Special Issues for Women

RADIATION

The tissue inside the vagina is delicate and sensitive to radiation. Pelvic radiation and cavitary implant therapy in the vagina or uterus can affect the physical structure and consistency of the vaginal mucosa (lining). These changes from radiation can cause discomfort during intercourse and internal pelvic examination. If you are not having regular weekly intercourse, please discuss vaginal dilators with a women's health clinician. Vaginal dilators are simple to use and help prevent the estrogen-deprived vaginal tissue from sticking together and collapsing in on itself. Vaginal dryness and changes in the acid/base balance in the vagina can make you more prone to yeast infections and urinary tract infections. See *Urination Problems*, p. 206, for remedies for UTIs. As for vaginal dryness, there are a number of good vaginal lubricants and moisturizers available. Replens, Astroglide, and Surgilube are all fine to use, depending on your personal preference. We do not recommend petroleum jelly, mineral oil, or any product that is not specifically intended for vaginal use. We recommend that you use these lubricants daily, as well as for vaginal intercourse, applying with a vaginal applicator or finger.

CONVENTIONAL MEDICATIONS

Viagra It is not known whether Viagra works for women. We do know that it is expensive and often not covered by insurance carriers. Viagra is also not recommended for people with cardiac or vascular problems. Viagra can also interact with many other medications. As of the time of this writing, Viagra is considered fairly controversial for use by women to improve sexual function.

HERBAL REMEDIES

Aphrodisiacs Ginger, cinnamon, cardamom, and anise—yes, these common spices have long been considered aphrodisiacs. Don't ingest large quantities of any of these herbs, but try a cup of spicy tea made with a few of these ingredients and see what happens. Ginger is not recommended for two days before surgery or together with other anticoagulants (feverfew, garlic, ginkgo, ginger, ginseng).

Calendula Cream This cream, made from the calendula flower, can be used as an effective vaginal moisturizer.

Chaste Tree Berry Although the name of this herb suggests it would inhibit desire, chaste tree berry (Vitex agnus castus) has been used to treat loss of libido in both women and men. A common dosage is 20 milligrams per day, usually taken in the form of a tincture (liquid extract). If you are taking oral contraceptives or are on hormone replacement therapy, we don't recommend taking this herb.

Dong Quai This herb (Angelica sinensis), used in traditional Chinese medicine, is considered an overall sexual tonic for women. You can take dong quai in capsules or tinctures. We recommend seeing a Chinese medicine practitioner for more information and specific dosing instructions. Be advised that in high dosages, people have experienced skin rashes and stomach upsets from this herb. It is not recommended that you take dong quai if you have diarrhea.

FERTILITY, PREGNANCY, AND BIRTH CONTROL

A woman's fertility can be seriously affected by cancer treatment. After having treatment with certain chemotherapies called alkylating agents (see below), women over thirty-five have an increased chance of experiencing premature menopause. For more information on premature menopause caused by chemotherapy, see *Menopause*, p. 153.

Alkylating Agents
- Carmustine (BiCNU, BCNU)
- Cisplatin (Cis-Platinum, CDDP, Platinol)
- Cyclophaosphamide (Cytoxan)
- Dacarbarzine (DTIC—Dome)
- Estamustine phosphate (Estracyte, Emcyt)
- Ifosfamide (IFEX)
- Lomustine (CCNU)
- Mechlorethamine hydrochloride (nitrogen mustard)
- Melphalan
- Streptozocin
- Thiotepa
- Nitrosomes

Ovaries and Radiation The ovaries are very sensitive to radiation therapy, so if one or both of your ovaries are in the radiation field, you will most likely go into premature menopause and become infertile. This is especially true for women who get total body irradiation (TBI) during the process of bone marrow transplant.

Amenorrhea Amenorrhea (the absence of your menstrual period) can occur for many reasons, including stress and weight loss, as well as from the cancer treatments discussed above. However, experiencing amenorrhea does not always mean that a woman is infertile.

> *If there is any possibility that you are pregnant before or during treatment, we urge you to discuss this with your clinician as soon as possible.*

Even if you believe that you will go into menopause because of the type of cancer treatment you receive, you should still use a reliable birth control method to prevent pregnancy while you are on treatment. Generally a woman is considered to be in menopause when she has had amenorrhea for three years or if the lack of certain hormones has been confirmed by blood tests.

Pregnancy Pregnancy during cancer treatment is generally not recommended due to the metabolic stress that pregnancy can put on a woman's body. It is advised that you wait for at least six months after your cancer treatment is completed to attempt getting pregnant. We strongly urge you to discuss any plans for pregnancy with your clinician. While there is no study that has proven that the incidence of birth defects increases after cancer treatment, if you are concerned, you should definitely seek the counsel of a cancer geneticist.

Special Issues for Men

DIAGNOSIS AND TREATMENT CONSIDERATIONS

Chemotherapy, hormone ablation therapy for prostate cancer—biclutamide (Casodex), estramustine (Emcyl), goserelin (Zoladex), and leuprolide (Lupron)—surgery, and radiation to the lower abdominal and pelvic area can all affect male sexuality. It is not at all uncommon for men to experience some degree of erectile dysfunction after cancer treatment, especially if this has been a problem before the cancer was diagnosed. This dysfunction can be short term or long term. In some men, testosterone production slows after pelvic radiation. However, these levels usually return to normal within six months after radiation therapy. Although this can be an embarrassing topic, we encourage you to speak openly to your clinician about any sexual problems you may be experiencing, as there may be medical treatments available that can help you. Depending on your individual problem, some of the options available to you are the prescription drug sildenafil (Viagra), vacuum constriction devices (a pump placed over the penis that draws blood into erectile tissue), penile injections (drugs injected directly into the side of the penis to help with erection), and permanent penile implants.

Speak with your clinician to help determine what's right for you and your specific problem. We recommend that you consider starting with the least invasive procedure first. Professional counseling and sex therapy can also be helpful to deal with anxiety regarding sexual function.

FERTILITY

Men have somewhat fewer long-term problems with fertility, as long as sperm production has not been affected by cancer treatment. However, despite this, you are still advised not to attempt pregnancy with your partner for at least six months after your treatment is completed.

RECOMMENDATIONS WHILE ON CANCER TREATMENT

It is highly recommended that you or your partner use condoms for sexual intercourse if you are in cancer treatment. This will prevent pregnancy and also prevent your partner from being exposed to minute amounts of systemic cancer treatment that may be present in your ejaculate for at least forty-eight hours after your chemotherapy infusion.

While on radiation treatment for prostate cancer, men are advised to avoid ejaculation, to prevent irritation to the internal treatment field.

FOR FURTHER INFORMATION

The organization Cancer Care has a sexuality and cancer program. On their website, www.cancercare.org, you can find information on prostate cancer and sexuality, as well as breast cancer and sexuality. To speak with a Cancer Care social worker, call Cancer Care at (212) 302-2400.

The American Cancer Society also has a wonderful website with information on sexuality and cancer for both men and women. See www2.cancer.org/patientguides for more information.

For more information on Viagra, you can visit the website www.viagra.com, which is sponsored by Pfizer, the pharmaceutical manufacturer of Viagra.

Oncolink also has a section on their website on sexuality and cancer; visit www.oncolink.upenn.edu/psychosocial for more information.

For more information on the complementary remedies discussed in this section, see chapter 3.

STRESS

A cancer diagnosis is stress provoking. While these feelings of stress are inevitable, how you deal with stress remains in your control.

Stress is the body's response to demands and pressures, both external and internal. Stress can be experienced as fatigue, irritability, or a general feeling of being overwhelmed. Imagine the feeling you experience when you are caught in an unexpected traffic jam and you needed to be somewhere ten minutes ago. That feeling is stress.

Disease and Treatment Considerations

ADRENOCORTICOIDS

If you need to take an adrenocorticoid (cortisone, hydrocortisone, dexamethasone, methyl prednisone, methyl prednisolone, prednisone, prednisilone) for treatment and/or symptom management, you may be experiencing feelings of stress as a side effect of the medication. If you believe your stress is related to one of these medications, discuss this possibility with your clinicians, as they may be able to modify your dose. However, you should *never* stop taking an oral steroid medication without guidance and supervision from your clinician.

THE IMPORTANCE OF DEALING WITH STRESS

Stress can affect your ability to heal. It can also alter the functioning of your immune system, making you more vulnerable to infection. In one study of breast cancer patients, those with the most anxiety about their diagnosis had the lowest levels of white blood cells. If you are starting to feel stressed while reading this, remember that there are things you can do to alter your stress level.

Some daily stress is necessary for living. Biologically speaking, even waking up in the morning is the result of a hormone-induced stress response. You are fasting while you are sleeping, so your initial feeling of hunger upon awaking is a stressor that helps you to wake up to eat.

Prevention

IDENTIFY THE STRESSES IN YOUR LIFE

If certain people and activities leave you feeling drained, stay away from them as much as possible. This may be a good time to reevaluate some situations in your life (relationships, work commitments, family issues) and be ruthless about eliminating negative influences. A diagnosis of cancer can be a reminder that you are precious and don't have the time to deal with unproductive situations or negative people.

Don't be afraid to admit that the stress you are feeling is real.

Talk to someone—a friend, a counselor, a hotline—and feel some relief when you let go of some of this burden.

> *Give yourself the gift of time for yourself, even an hour, to listen to music you love, take a yoga class, write in a journal, or watch the clouds go by.*

- Do a stress-reducing activity such as walking, dancing, listening to music, or taking a soothing bubble bath. (See *Relaxation,* p. 252.)
- Support your metabolic energy by eating enough calories, drinking enough fluids, and trying to incorporate a little physical movement into your routine every day. If your energy bank is in a depleted condition, it will be harder to manage stress.
- Make sure your sleep is restful. See *Sleep Problems,* p. 192, for suggestions on improving the quality of sleep.
- Learn to say no, and leave it at that, when you don't feel like doing something.

Remedies

For stressful events that you can't control, such as your medical treatments, traffic jams, or family issues, try to use relaxation methods to deal with the stress. See *Relaxation,* p. 252, and *Meditation,* p. 242, for suggestions.

ASK FOR HELP

Many people with cancer and other chronic diseases feel that they have to cope with everything all by themselves. Remember that you are not alone. There are organizations out there designed to help cancer patients deal with the stress of diagnosis. Your clinician may be able to refer you to a social worker who can help you with all sorts of problems. You owe it to yourself to avail yourself of these resources.

DON'T BLAME YOURSELF

One significant source of stress for some cancer patients is a belief that they are somehow responsible for their diagnosis. We can't emphasize enough the fallacy of this idea. You are not to blame for your cancer. No one knows exactly what causes cancer. Cancer is most likely a complicated interaction involving a number of factors. What we do know is that feeling responsible for getting the disease is only going to create stress and won't help to promote your healing.

AROMATHERAPY

Take a relaxing warm bath with an essential oil that you find calming. Try chamomile, lavender, or sandalwood oil.

BACH FLOWER REMEDIES

Aspen—for dealing with anxiety and apprehension
Elm—for when you feel overwhelmed

OTHER WAYS TO REDUCE STRESS

· Don't put too much pressure on yourself.
· Set small daily goals that are achievable to prevent frustration and despair (see *Fatigue*, p. 122).
· Try to laugh as much as possible. Rent movies that make you laugh—the sillier the better.

VITAMINS

B-complex vitamins have been shown to reduce stress. However, you should not take folic acid or folate if you are on treatment for gastric, colon, or anal cancer. Folic acid is also not appropriate if you are getting methotrexate or leucovorin. Supplemental B_6 is not recommended if you are on cisplatin (Platinol) or carboplatin. Avoid taking these supplements for two days before and after the chemotherapy infusion.

WE DO NOT RECOMMEND

- Don't try to be stoic.
- Don't suppress or repress your feelings.
- Don't try to take care of everything and everybody by yourself. When people offer to help, make a note of it and call in the offers when you need them.

For Further Information

The website www.calmcentre.com is dedicated to enhancing feelings of calm. Enter the meditation room and watch a cloud float across your screen for an instant meditation experience.

For more information on the complementary remedies discussed in this section, see chapter 3.

WIGS

Hair loss during cancer treatment can be a very upsetting side effect for both men and women (see *Hair Loss*, p. 130). This section is intended to apply to both men and women, as the recommendations regarding the purchase, fit, and styling of wigs also apply to hairpieces.

Radiation

If you are getting radiation to the head, discuss with your radiation therapist during your treatment planning where you are most likely to lose hair. This will help you determine how you would like to manage this problem—with a wig, a hairpiece, restyling, or a hat.

> *If your hair loss is not severe or you don't wish to buy a wig, a sensitive hairstylist can make a world of difference in your appearance.*

Purchasing a Wig

If you want to purchase a wig, here are some tips.

FINANCIAL CONSIDERATIONS

Try to determine whether your health insurance will cover the cost of a wig. If your insurance does not cover this, you can try contacting the customer service department of your health insurance company to find out if calling a wig a "hair prosthesis" would make a difference. Ask your clinician to provide you with a prescription for a "hair prosthesis" to get the cost covered. Besides insurance, there are other sources of financial aid for wigs (or hair prostheses). If you are eligible, go ahead and apply. Your clinicians should have information about this; if not, call your local chapter of the American Cancer Society. Some hospitals and cancer centers have wigs that have been donated by former clients or good Samaritans.

FINDING A WIG

Do you have a regular hair cutter or stylist? Ask them if they can recommend a wig store. Some salons have an employee or colleague who specializes in wig care. We have found that the Internet is another good source for wig information. You may be amazed at how many wigs are available and how many choices you may have. The American Cancer Society, at (800) ACS-2345 or www.cancer.org, provides a list of wig stores that cater to cancer survivors.

BEFORE YOU BUY A WIG

Once you find a wig that you like, don't immediately buy it. See if you can order the wig or put it on hold. Go home and think about this wig. Go to a couple of other stores and see what else is available. Remember that wig selling is a business and you are the customer, so only buy what you like on your head.

When you go to find a wig, we recommend that you go with a trusted friend or family member. Remember, the goal of a wig is to help you look like yourself. Now is not necessarily the time to try a new color or an outrageous style, although if you also want a wig that is pure fun, there's nothing wrong with indulging yourself. The store should have good lighting and lots of well-placed mirrors so that you don't have to guess what the wig really looks like. Bring an instant camera such as a Polaroid if you can, and take pictures of your entire head, so you will know what you look like from the back. This way you can look at the pictures before you buy the wig.

SHOPPING FOR A WIG

Try to go to a wig store while you still have your hair so that the color and texture of your natural hair can be matched as closely as possible to the wig. Wig stores are generally a true specialty. Call first to make an appointment to meet the wig fitters and have a consultation. If you are uncomfortable in the shop or the person helping you is not a good match for you, move on.

Remember that it is the rare wig that does not need to be restyled after purchase. A sensitive stylist can make all the difference in your appearance.

CONSIDERATIONS TO KEEP IN MIND

Wigs can be expensive and look awful. Conversely, they can be relatively inexpensive and look terrific. We have found, generally speaking, that brunette wigs often can fall in the inexpensive, terrific-looking category. It certainly helps to consider who are the groups of people who buy wigs and learn where they shop. There are some groups (Jewish orthodox, Caribbean, and African-American, for example), where women are more likely to wear wigs and hairpieces. Stores that cater to these groups can be very helpful resources to you. Remember, it is not the price but the appearance that is important. No one has to know how little this wig cost except you. Remember, too, that the wig is to help you get through the temporary loss of hair. It is not likely to be permanent.

Wigs can be uncomfortable, especially in hot and humid climates and seasons. It is possible to wear a "liner" between your scalp and the wig, but it keeps the heat in. Some people wear a wig at certain times and not at others. We recommend that you think about these issues before you invest in a wig. Some people buy a wig but decide not to wear it because they find it uncomfortable. If you are unsure, you don't have to spend a lot of money. You can buy a trial wig first before making a big purchase.

HUMAN HAIR WIGS

Usually the most expensive wigs are those made of human hair. Be aware that human hair wigs require good and consistent care. If they are not cared for well, human hair wigs have a tendency to look dull and limp. Like your own hair, human hair wigs require proper care and attention (see below for care instructions). Unlike your own hair, however, human hair wigs should not be slept in or worn in bed for long periods of time, as they mat very easily. There are also wigs with a combination of human and synthetic hair.

CAN EVERYONE TELL?

The answer is NO. There are many people out there who hear the words "cancer treatment" and assume that you are wearing a wig—which can be very amusing when you are not. Of course, if you are wearing a wig and have become more knowledgeable about wigs, you tend to notice them more frequently on others. We believe this is because you are more educated and aware of wigs, not because the wigs themselves are that noticeable. However, a bad wig is a bad wig. Sometimes a wig is more noticeable because it needs to be cleaned and restyled; sometimes it doesn't fit properly. That is why we feel it is important to buy a wig with someone you know—someone who has no problem at all telling you what the wig really looks like on your head.

CARE AND STYLING FOR YOUR WIG

Washing a wig is very similar to hand washing a good wool sweater. The key is to be gentle. Wigs, like clothing, come with care instructions. Be sure to check the wig manufacturer's recommendations for the proper wig care. For best results, we recommend that you have your wig professionally cut and styled.

HOW OFTEN TO WASH YOUR WIG

Wash your wig as often as it needs to be washed, but we don't recommend washing it more frequently than every seven to ten days if you are wearing it every day. If you need your wig every day, consider buying two wigs so you can rotate them. Washing and styling can take two full days to allow proper drying.

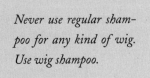

Never use regular shampoo for any kind of wig. Use wig shampoo.

WASHING YOUR WIG

For non-human-hair wigs, dissolve a capful of synthetic wig shampoo or a mild soap like Woolite in a basin of cool water (this protects curls). For a human-hair wig, use a human-hair wig shampoo in lukewarm water. If your wig has picked up odors (smoke, perfume, etc.), add a tea-spoon of baking soda to the water.

Submerge the wig gently until it is saturated by the water and shampoo. Gently scrub the area of the wig that meets your forehead to loosen skin oil residue on the wig lining. Let the wig soak for about fif-teen minutes. Never twist water out of a wig; just squeeze the water out gently. Spread your wig out on a towel and air dry overnight. You can also clip your wig to a hanger to dry.

After the wig is completely dry (usually after two days in the air), use a hair dryer on a low setting. You can spray on wig conditioner if you wish to restyle with your fingers, but *never* use a curling iron on a syn-thetic hair wig. You can use a curling iron on a human hair wig; how-ever, if you want to restyle in a more elaborate style, put the wig on a stand and use rollers, papers, and pins. Spray ice water to wet the pinned hair and style as you desire. Let the wig air dry again overnight.

If all this wig care feels like too much work, ask your hairstylist if he or she does wig care. We recommend that you ask the cost of the serv-ice before agreeing to it.

Look Good, Feel Better

The American Cancer Society also has a wonderful program called Look Good, Feel Better, which is a one-time hair and makeup session for women. This program is free, and you must sign up in advance. These sessions are reported to be a lot of fun, and women find them very good sources of practical information on things like wigs, head coverings, and appearance. You can find more information at www.lookgoodfeelbetter.org or by calling your local ACS chapter.

Unfortunately, there is not yet an equivalent to the Look Good, Feel Better program for men, although we believe there should be. If you are so motivated—start one and let us know how it goes. We'd love to hear about it.

For more information on the complementary remedies discussed in this section, see chapter 3.

In Conclusion

There are some things we would like you to be able to take away from this book. Although neither of us has personally had the experience of cancer, we have known and loved at least one person in our lives who has. What have we learned from them? Everything we have included in this book and more. But the most important thing we have learned is that life is precious, and to experience life to its fullest it must be lived in the present moment. We encourage you to embrace your life and live it well.

Our intention in writing this book was to provide information and present options to help you make some very difficult decisions. We hope that you have found our explanations of symptoms and their solutions helpful and are now aware of many remedy options you didn't know you had. We know that there is a vast array of information and there are many more choices out there than we could possibly cover in a single book. That is why we have tried to provide you with the tools and resources for making your own decisions and for seeking out more information when you need it. Ultimately, it is your life, and no one else can make decisions for you.

We would also like to remind you that even if your clinicians are pushing you to make fast decisions, you always have a little time to think things over and weigh your options. If you feel that a decision you have made is not working for you, change it. It is a very rare case where you cannot change your mind and do something else.

All of us will eventually live with some kind of health problem; the difference will be in how we each choose to live with it. We wrote this book to help you live well because, after all, living well is the best revenge.

All the best,
Katen Moore and Libby Schmais

Resources

BOOKS

American Cancer Society's Guide to Complementary and Alternative Cancer Methods. Atlanta: American Cancer Society, 2000.

Balch, James, and Phyllis A. Balch. *Prescription for Nutritional Healing.* New York: Avery, 1998.

Boik, John. *Cancer and Natural Medicine: A Textbook of Basic Science and Clinical Research.* Princeton, MN: Oregon Medical Press, 1996.

Brinker, Francis. *Herb Contraindications and Drug Interactions.* Sandy, OR: Eclectic Medical Publications, 1998.

Bruning, Nancy. *Coping with Chemotherapy.* New York: Ballantine, 1993.

Cancer Care, Inc. *A Helping Hand.* New York: Cancer Care Inc., 1998.

Christensen, Alice. *The American Yoga Association Beginner's Manual.* New York: Simon and Schuster, 1987.

Coleman, Norman. *Understanding Cancer: A Patient's Guide to Diagnosis, Prognosis and Treatment.* John Hopkins University Press, 1998.

Decker, Georgia M., ed. *An Introduction to Complementary and Alternative Therapies.* Pittsburgh: Oncology Nursing Press, 1999.

DeVita, V. T., S. Hellman, and S. A. Rosenberg. *Cancer: Principles and Practice of Oncology.* Philadelphia: Lippincott-Raven, 1997.

Dodd, Marilyn J. *Managing the Side Effects of Chemotherapy and Radiation Therapy: A Guide for Patients and Their Families.* San Francisco: UCSF Nursing Press, 1996.

Editors of Time-Life Books. *The Medical Advisor: The Complete Guide to Alternative and Conventional Treatments.* Alexandria, VA: Time-Life, 1997.

Fischbach, Frances. *A Manual of Laboratory and Diagnostic Tests.* Philadelphia: Lippin-cott-Raven, 1996.

Gach, M.R. *Acupressure's Potent Points.* New York: Bantam, 1990.

Garrison, Robert, Jr., and Elizabeth Somer. *The Nutrition Desk Reference.* New York: Keats, 1995.

Goleman, D., and J. Gurin, eds. *Mind/Body Medicine: How to Use Your Mind for Better Health.* Yonkers, NY: Consumers Union of the United States, 1993.

Gottlieb, Bill, ed. *New Choices in Natural Healing.* New York: Rodale Press, 1995.

Graedon, Joe, and Teresa Graedon. *The People's Pharmacy.* New York: St. Martin's Press, 1998.

Haller, James. *What to Eat When You Don't Feel Like Eating.* Hansport, Nova Scotia: Lancelot Press Limited, 1994.

Harpham, Wendy Schlessel. *Diagnosis: Cancer.* New York: Norton, 1997.

Heimbeurger, D. C., and R. L. Weinsier. *Handbook of Clinical Nutrition.* St. Louis: Mosby, 1997.

Kenyon, J. *Acupressure Techniques: A Self-Help Guide.* Rochester, VT: Healing Arts Press, 1988.

Kloss, Jethro. *Back to Eden.* Loma Linda: Back to Eden, 1992.

Krieger, Dolores K. *Therapeutic Touch.* New York: Simon and Schuster, 1994.

Lerner, Michael. *Choices in Healing.* Boston: MIT Press, 1996.

LeShan, Lawrence. *How to Meditate: A Guide to Self-Discovery.* New York: Bantam Books, 1984.

Link, John. *The Breast Cancer Survival Manual.* New York: Owl Books, 1998.

Miller, Lucinda G., and Wallace J. Murray, eds. *Herbal Medicinals.* Binghamton, NY: Haworth Press, 1998.

Northrup, Christiane. *Women's Bodies, Women's Wisdom.* New York: Bantam Books, 1998.

Nuland, Sherwin B. *How We Die: Reflections on Life's Final Chapter.* New York: Knopf, 1994.

Peirce, Andrea. *The American Pharmaceutical Association Practical Guide to Natural Med-icines.* New York: Morrow, 1999.

Rippin, Joanna. *Aromatherapy for Health, Relaxation and Well-Being.* New York: Lorenz Books, 1997.

Sandifer, J. *Acupressure for Health, Vitality and First Aid.* Rockport, MA: Element Press, 1997.

Schultz, V., R. Hansel, and V. E. Tyler. *Rational Phytotherapy: A Physicans' Guide to Herbal Medication.* Berlin, Germany: Springer-Verlag, 1998.

Sifton, David, ed. *The PDR Family Guide to Natural Medicines and Healing Therapies.* New York: Three Rivers Press, 1999.

Simon, David. *Return to Wholeness.* New York: Wiley, 1999.

Smith, Jean, ed. *Breath Sweeps Mind: A First Guide to Meditation Practice.* New York: Riverhead Books, 1998.

Tobin, Daniel. *Peaceful Dying: The Step-by-Step Guide to Preserving Your Dignity, Your Choice, and Your Inner Peace at the End of Life.* Reading, MA: Perseus Books, 1999.

Tyler, Varro E., and James E. Robbers. *The Therapeutic Use of Phytomedicinals.* Bing-hamton, NY: Haworth Press, 1998.

Tyler, Varro E., and Steven Foster. *The Honest Herbal.* Binghamton, NY: Haworth Press, 1998.

Ullman, Dana. *The Consumer's Guide to Homeopathy.* New York: Putnam, 1995.

Weed, Susun. *Breast Cancer? Breast Health! The Wise Woman Way.* Woodstock, NY: Ash Tree Publishing, 1997.

Weil, Andrew. *Natural Health, Natural Medicine.* Boston: Houghton Mifflin, 1998.

Whitaker, Julian. *Dr. Whitaker's Guide to Natural Healing.* Rocklin, CA: Prima, 1996.

Wilkes, G. M., K. Ingwerson, and M. B. Burke. *2000 Oncology Nursing Drug Handbook.* Sudbury, MA: Jones and Bartlett, 1999.

Worwood, Valerie Ann. *The Complete Book of Essential Oils and Aromatherapy.* San Rafael: New World Library, 1991.

ARTICLES

Austin, Steve. 1998. B12 Deficiency: A possible nutritional link to urinary incontinence. *Quarterly Review of Natural Medicine.* (15 December): 305.

Bottiglieri, T., K. Hyland, and E. H. Reynolds. 1994. The clinical potential of ademethionine (S-adenosylmethionine) in neurological disorders. *Drugs* 48(2): 137–52.

Bove, G., and N. Nilsson. 1998. Spinal manipulation in the treatment of episodic tension-type headache. *JAMA* 280: 1576–79.

Cancer patients try many forms of alternative therapy. 1997. *Cancer Weekly Plus.* August 11, 1997: 6–7.

Davis, L., and G. Kuttan. 1998. Suppressive effect of cyclophosphamide induced toxicity by Withania somnifera extract in mice. *Journal of Ethnopharmacology* 62: 209–14.

Dibble, S. L., et al. Acupressure for nausea: Results of a pilot study. *Oncology Nursing Forum* 27(1): 41–47.

Dundee, J. W., et al. 1989. Nausea, vomiting and postoperative pain. *British Journal of Anesthesia* 63(5): 612–18.

Duvic, M. 1996. A randomized trial of minoxidil in chemotherapy-induced alopecia. *Journal of the American Academy of Dermatology* 35: 84–87.

Fava, M., et al. 1995. Rapidity of onset of the antidepressant effect of parenteral S-adenosyl-L-methioninine. *Psychiatry Research* 56(3): 295–97.

Ferrell-Torry, A. T., and O. J. Glick. 1993. The use of therapeutic massage as a nursing intervention to modify anxiety and the perception of cancer pain. *Cancer Nursing* 16(2): 93–101.

Hammar, M., J. Frisk, O. Grimas, M. Hook, A. C. Spetz, and Y. Wyon. 1999. Acupuncture treatment of vasomotor symptoms in men with prostatic carcinoma: A pilot study. *Journal of Urology* 161(3): 853–56.

Hay, I. C., M. Jamieson, and A. D. Ormerod. 1998. Randomized trial of aromatherapy: Successful treatment for alopecia areata. *Archives of Dermatology* 134(11): 1349–52.

Hobbs, Christopher. 1997. Mushroom medicine. *Vegetarian Times* 243: 96–99.

Khalsa, Dharma Singh. 1998. Integrated Medicine and the prevention and reversal of memory loss. *Alternative Therapies in Health and Medicine* 4(6): 38–43.

Levy, M. H. 1992 (reprint). Constipation and diarrhea in cancer patients. *Cancer Bulletin* 43(5): 412–22.

Linde, K., et al. 1997. Are the clinical effects of homeopathy placebo effects? A meta-analysis of placebo-controlled trials. *Lancet* 351: 220.

Living with cancer, don't go it alone. *Harvard Health Letter*, May 9, 1997.

Mills, E. E. 1988. The modifying effect of beta-carotene on radiation and chemotherapy induced oral mucositis. *British Journal of Cancer* 57: 416–17.

Mock, V., et al. 1997. Effects of exercise on fatigue, physical functioning, and emotional distress during radiation therapy for breast cancer. *Oncology Nursing Forum* 24(6): 991–1000.

Nakano, H., et al. 1999. A multi-institutional prospective study of lentinan in advanced gastric cancer patients with unresectable and recurrent disease: Effect on prolongation of survival and improvement of quality of life. *Hepatogastroenterology* 46(28): 2662–68.

Pickard-Holley, S. 1995. The symptom experience of alopecia. *Seminar in Oncology Nursing* 11: 235–38.

Richardson, M. A., et al. 1997. Coping, life attitudes and immune responses to imagery and group support after breast cancer treatment. *Alternative Therapies in Health and Medicine* 3(5): 62–70.

Ripamonti, C., et al. 1998. A randomized, controlled clinical trial to evaluate the effects of zinc sulfate on cancer patients with taste alterations caused by head and neck irradiation. *Cancer* 82(10): 1938–45.

Schempp, C. M., et al. 1999. Antibacterial activity of Hyperforin from St. John's Wort against multiresistant staphylococcus, aures and gram-positive bacteria. *Lancet* 353: 21–29.

Scherer, J. 1998. Kava-kava extract in anxiety disorders: An outpatient observational study. *Advances in Therapy* 15: 261–69.

Schmidt, G., and D. Soyka. 1994. Effect of peppermint and eucalyptus oil preparations on neurophysiological and experimental algesimetric headache parameters. *Cephalgia* 14(3): 228–34.

Schulick, Paul. 1996. The healing power of ginger. *Vegetarian Times* (May): 78–83.

Spiegel, D. 1996. Cancer and depression. *British Journal of Psychiatry* 168: 109–16.

Stengler, Mark. 1998. Supplements and chemotherapy. *Nature's Impact* (November): 53.

Tate, S., et al. 1997. Peppermint oil: A treatment for postoperative nausea. *Journal of Advanced Nursing* 26(3): 543–49.

U.S. FDA considers effects of maitake mushroom in treating cancer. *Cancer Weekly Plus*, March 1, 1999.

Wadleigh, R.G., et al. 1992. Vitamin E in the treatment of chemotherapy-induced mucositis. *American Journal of Medicine* 92(5): 481–84.

Weber, Susan, Volkman Nuessler, and Wolfgang Wilmanns. 1997. A pilot study on the influence of receptive music listening on cancer patients during chemotherapy. *International Journal of Arts Medicine* 5(2): 27–35.

Wilkes, G. 2000. Nutrition: The forgotten ingredient in cancer care. *American Journal of Nursing* 100(4): 46–51.

Winstead-Fry, P., and J. Kijek. 1999. An integrative review and meta-analysis of therapeutic touch research. *Alternative Therapies in Health and Medicine* 5(6): 58–67.

Ziauddin, M., et al. 1996. Studies on the immunomodulatory effects of ashwagandha. *Journal of Ethnopharmacology* 50: 69–76.

JOURNALS, MAGAZINES, AND NEWSLETTERS

Advance for Nurse Practitioners. King of Prussia, PA: Merion Publications.
American Journal of Nursing. Washington, D.C.: American Nursing Association.
Clinical Journal of Oncology Nursing. Pittsburgh, PA: Oncology Nursing Press.
Herbalgram. Austin, TX: American Botanical Council and Herb Research Foundation.
Integrative Medicine Consult. Newburgh, NY: Integrative Medicine Communications.
Mamm. New York: Poz Publishing.
Natural Health. Boston: Weider Publishing.
Oncology Nursing Forum. Pittsburgh, PA: Oncology Nursing Press.
Prevention Magazine. New York: Rodale Press.

ORGANIZATIONS

American Alliance of Aromatherapy
PO Box 750428
Petaluma, CA 94975-0428

American Aromatherapy Association
PO Box 3679
South Pasadena, CA 91031
www.aromaweb.com

American Association of Acupuncture and Oriental Medicine
433 Front Street
Catasauqua, PA 18032
(610) 266-1433
Fax: (610) 264-2768
www.aaom.org

Provides referrals to qualified professional acupuncturists and practitioners of Chinese medicine.

American Botanical Council
PO Box 201660
Austin, TX 78720
(512) 926-4900
www.herbalgram.org

Provides information on herbs and other dietary supplements.

American Cancer Society
www.cancer.org
(800) ACS-2345

Provides information to patients on cancer treatment, early detection, and prevention, as well as information on a variety of services available to cancer patients and their families.

American Chiropractic Association
1701 Clarendon Blvd.
Arlington, VA 22209
(703) 276-8800
Fax: (703) 243-2593
www.amerchiro.org

Provides information about chiropractic and where to find a chiropractor in your area.

American Massage Therapy Association
820 Davis Street, Suite 100
Evanston, IL 60201-4444
(847) 864-0123
www.amtamassage.org

Provides information on massage therapy and choosing a therapist.

American Self-Help Clearinghouse
(201) 625-7101

American Society of Clinical Hypnosis
2200 East Vine Avenue, Suite 291
Des Plaines, IL 60018
(630) 980-4740
www.asch.net

Provides information and referrals to hypnotists.

American Society of Clinical Oncology
225 Reinekers Lane, Suite 650
Alexandria, VA 22314-2875
(703) 299-0150
www.asco.org

Provides information on treatment choices.

American Yoga Association
PO Box 19986
Sarasota, FL 34276
(941) 927-4977
www.members.aol.com/amyogaassn

Another good place to buy yoga tapes, books, and accessories is the website of the magazine *Yoga Journal* at www.yogajournal.com.

Association of Cancer Online Resources
www.acor.org

Hosts and manages a large number of cancer-specific online information resources and support groups.

Dr. Edward Bach Foundation
The Bach Centre
Mount Vernon
Bakers Lane, Sotwell
Oxon, OX10 0PZ, UK
Telephone: +44 (0) 1491 834678
Fax: +44 (0) 1491 825022
www.bachcentre.com

Bio-Electro-Magnetics Institute
2490 West Moana Lane
Reno, NV 89509-3936
(775) 827-9099

Cancercare
www.cancercare.org

Cancer Hope Network
www.cancerhopenetwork.org

This not-for-profit organization provides free one-on-one support with trained volunteers to cancer patients and their families.

Cancer-Info
www.cancer-info.com

An online chat and news forum for cancer patients, families, and professionals.

Cancer Supportive Care Programs
www.cancersupportivecare.com

This site contains supportive care information on topics that include nutrition, fatigue, anemia, pain control, and lymphedema.

Cansearch: A Guide to Cancer Resources on the Internet
www.cansearch.org/cansearch/canserch.htm

Cansearch is produced by the National Coalition for Cancer Survivorship (NCCS) to provide survivors and patients with a step-by-step guide to the many cancer resources found on the Web.

The Center for Mind Body Medicine
5225 Connecticut Avenue NW, Suite 414

Washington, D.C. 20015
(202) 966-7338
www.cmbm.org

CMBM is a wonderful organization committed to transforming the practice of medicine and reviving the spirit.

Choice in Dying
1035 30th Street NW
Washington, D.C. 20007
(202) 338-9790
Fax: (202) 338-0242
www.choices.org

Provides information and legal counseling on end-of-life decisions.

Commonweal Cancer Project
PO Box 316
Bolinas, CA 94924
(415) 868-0970
Fax: (415) 868-2230
www.commonweal.org

Provides support for people with cancer; emphasizes integrating conventional with complementary treatment.

Corporate Angel Network
www.corpangelnetwork.org

The Corporate Angel Network (CAN) provides cancer patients with free air transportation to and from medical facilities by using empty seats on corporate aircraft. Patients must meet CAN's qualifications but do not need to meet any financial-need criteria.

Food and Nutrition Information Center
USDA-National Agricultural Library
10301 Baltimore Avenue, Room 304
Beltsville, MD 20705-2351
(301) 504-5719
www.nal.usda.gov/fnic/

Provides materials, information, and library on general nutrition, including resources on nutrition and cancer.

Gilda's Club
www.gildasclub.org

Gilda's Clubs provide supportive services to cancer patients and their families. Lectures, workshops, networking groups, special events, and a children's program are available.

Healthfinder
www.healthfinder.gov

The U.S. Department of Health and Human Services offers this free gateway to consumer health information.

Herb Research Foundation
1007 Pearl Street, Suite 200
Boulder, CO 80302
(303) 449-2265
www.herbs.org

Provides information on herbal remedies, research, regulatory issues, and general information.

Hospice Foundation of America
www.hospicefoundation.org
1-800-854-3402

The Leukemia & Lymphoma Society
www.leukemia.org
New York City Chapter
475 Park Avenue South, 21st Floor
New York, NY 10016
(800) 955-4572

Look Good, Feel Better
The American Cancer Society
1-800-ACS-2345
www.lookgoodfeelbetter.org

Teaches women who have undergone cancer treatment how to improve their appearance with cosmetics, wigs, and scarves.

Dr. Susan Love (author of *Dr. Susan Love's Breast Book*)
www.susanlovemd.com

Meditation Center
www.meditationcenter.com
A good meditation resource.

National Cancer Institute Cancer Information Service/PDQ
9000 Rockville Pike
Bethesda, MD 20982
1- 800-4-CANCER
www.cancernet.nci.nih.gov

Provides current, comprehensive information on all major types of cancer, treatments, and clinical trials.

National Center for Homeopathy
801 N. Fairfax Street, Suite 306
Alexandria, VA 22314
(703) 548-7790
www.homeopathic.org

Provides information on homeopathy and instructional programs.

National Commission for the Certification of Acupuncturists
(202) 232-1404

National Hospice Organization
1901 N. Moore Street, Suite 901
Arlington, VA 22209
(703) 243-5900
(800) 658-8898
www.nho.org

Provides information and referrals to local hospitals, patient advocacy, and professional education.

National Prostate Cancer Coalition
1300 19th Street NW, Suite 400
Washington, D.C. 20036
(202) 463-9455
www.4npcc.org

North American Menopause Society
PO Box 94527
Cleveland, OH 44101
(216) 844-8748
www.menopause.org

Nurse Healers Professional Associates
3760 South Highland Drive, Suite 429
Salt Lake City, UT 84106
(801) 273-3399
www.therapeutic-touch.org

OncoChat
www.oncochat.org

An online chat forum for cancer patients, families, and professionals.

Oncolink
oncolink.upenn.edu

Sponsored by the University of Pennsylvania, this website offers a comprehensive, well-organized source of cancer information for patients and healthcare professionals.

Patient Advocate Organization
www.patientadvocate.org

Provides education, legal counseling, and referrals to cancer patients and survivors concerning managed care, insurance, financial issues, job discrimination, and debt crisis matters.

PharmInfoNet
www.pharminfo.com
An online drug information resource.

PubMed
www.ncbi.nlm.nih.gov/PubMed/

Online search service accessing millions of citations in the National Library of Medicine's bibliographic database of journals published worldwide.

United Ostomy Association
19772 MacArthur Boulevard, Suite 200
Irvine, CA 92612
(800) 826-0826
www.uoa.org

Wellness Community
35 East 7th Street, Suite 412
Cincinnati, OH 45202
(513) 421-7111
www.wellness-community.org

This organization, similar to Gilda's Club, has sites around the country that provide emotional support and educational programs for cancer patients and their loved ones.

Y-Me WIG
212 West Van Buren Street, 4th Floor
Chicago, IL 60607
(800) 221-2141
Fax: (312) 294-8598
www.y-me.org

Provides donated wigs free of charge.

GLOSSARY

anemia   a symptom of disease or treatment where the amount and size of red blood cells are insufficient to meet the body's demand for oxygen.

blood counts   the numbers and types of blood cells counted from a 1-cubic-millimeter sample of blood.

breakthrough pain   pain or discomfort experienced despite being on a long-acting opioid, that requires additional short-acting or long-acting opioid for sufficient pain control.

chronic obstructive pulmonary disease (COPD)   any chronic process that interferes permanently with the lungs' ventilatory function, that is, emphysema.

coagulation   the state when a fluid has changed to a semisolid mass; used when referring to blood-clotting mechanisms.

compounding pharmacy   a specialty of pharmacy, used most often in pediatrics and hospice, that can help create medications that can be used via alternative routes than what they had been originally designed for; for example, making a suppository version of an oral medication or a transdermal patch of what is usually an oral or rectal medication.

cytoprotectant   a substance or process that protects cells.

cytotoxic   a substance or process that is toxic to cells.

diuresis   a process that triggers the vascular system to secrete large amounts of fluid as urine.

edema   tissue swelling from excessive amounts of fluid; can be caused by a variety of reasons related to inactivity and dependent limbs, tissue injury, after surgery, electrolyte imbalance, and so forth.

epidural catheter   a catheter that enters the epidural space in the spinal cord to allow direct pain control. Most often used for nerve block procedures with painful metastases to the back.

equianalgesic   a dose of one opioid that provides pain relief equilavent to the dose of another opioid; used to facilitate good pain management when switching opioids.

gut   the bowel or intestine.

hematocrit   the percentage of total blood volume that consists of red blood cells after the sample has been spun in a centrifuge and allowed to separate from the plasma.

hemoglobin   the protein in the red blood cell that carries oxygen from the lungs for use in the body's tissues; also contains iron.

infusion   the process of introducing a liquid therapeutic substance into the body intravenously.

local therapy   treatment at one specific site.

metastasis   the spread of a cancer from its primary site.

mucosa   the mucous membrane that lines a hollow organ or body cavity.

mucositis   inflammation of a mucous membrane. Most often used when describing inflammation in the mouth, throat, and esophagus due to radiation therapy or certain chemotherapies.

neurotoxic   a substance that is toxic to the nervous system.

neutropenia   the state of having too few neutrophils and therefore too few white blood cells to maintain adequate immune function.

neutrophils   the most common type of white blood cell and the most responsible for maintaining immune function.

nonsteroidal anti-inflammatory drugs (NSAIDs)   the class of medications similar to aspirin that have mild analgesic, anti-inflammatory, and antipyretic (fever) action. The short-acting NSAID ibuprofen is *generally* preferred for use for people with cancer.

paresthesias   numbness, tingling, burning sensation felt especially in the fingers, hands, toes, and feet.

phytoestrogens   estrogenlike chemicals found in plants; it is believed that they are metabolized differently from endogenous (the body's own) estrogen and therefore may be safe for those with estrogen-sensitive cancers.

platelets   a cell, found in the blood, that is critical to the coagulation process.

sedation   the state of being calmed.

subcutaneous injection   an injection of medication into the fatty layer just under the skin.

systemic therapy   treatment for the whole body, usually via infusion.

thrombocytopenia   the state of having too few platelets.

tolerance   when a dose of medication needs to be increased to produce the same effect without adverse side effects. Commonly experienced with prolonged use of opioid medications.

transdermal   a way to administer medication through the skin.

transfusion   the intravenous administration of a blood product.

INDEX

ABOUT THE AUTHORS

KATEN MOORE is a graduate of Barnard College and the MGH Institute of Health Professions at Massachusetts General Hospital. She currently works as an oncology clinical research nurse at Somerset Medical Center in New Jersey. Previously, Katen worked as an oncology nurse practitioner at Harvard Pilgrim Healthcare in Boston. Katen has conducted workshops in cancer wellness and grief intervention in New York, New Jersey, and Massachusetts. She lives with her husband, Kevin, and daughter, Aurelia, in New Jersey.

LIBBY SCHMAIS is a graduate of Clark University, Pratt Institute, and Brooklyn College. Libby currently works as a researcher and a freelance writer. Her first novel, *The Perfect Elizabeth* (July 2000), was published by St. Martin's Press and was chosen as part of the Barnes & Noble Discover Great New Writers Program. Libby lives in New York with her husband, Sam.